SWALLOWING
A BITTER PILL

SWALLOWING A BITTER PILL

*How Prescription and Over-the-counter
Drug Abuse is Ruining Lives
– My Story –*

Cindy R. Mogil

New Horizon Press
Far Hills, New Jersey

New Horizon Press
P.O. Box 669
Far Hills, NJ 07931

Cindy R. Mogil
    Swallowing A Bitter Pill: How Prescription and Over-the-counter Drug
    Abuse is Ruining Lives – My Story

Cover Design: Robert Aulicino
Interior Design: Susan M. Sanderson

Library of Congress Control Number: 2001089170

ISBN: 0-88282-211-X
New Horizon Press

Manufactured in the U.S.A.

2005   2004   2003   2002   2001 / 5   4   3   2   1

DEDICATION

To God, for granting me the *Courage* to admit that I am powerless over my addiction to pills and any mood-altering substances; the *Wisdom* that I have gained through support groups, my sponsor and prayer, so that I may share with others that still suffer; and the *Serenity* that comes from within that can be felt not only by me, but those I choose to have in my life.

To my husband, *Michael*, for his unconditional love, encouragement and support. Thank you for your inspiration and wisdom, always believing in me, trusting our love and believing in the miracle of recovery.

To my son, *Lucien*, for his sense of humor and ability to lift my spirits when I need it the most. I love you with all my heart and soul.

To *my family*, for their wisdom, love and support. God has blessed me with a family that has taught me to believe in myself and never give up what I know is right.

Author's Note

This book is based on my research and experiences with prescription and over-the-counter drug addiction and recovery, as well as the experiences of others struggling with this destructive disorder. In order to protect privacy, fictitious names and identities have been given to some individuals in this book and otherwise identifying characteristics have been altered. For the purposes of simplifying usage, the pronouns his/him and her are often used interchangeably.

The material in this book is intended to provide information and raise awareness about prescription addiction. This book serves only as a supplement to, not a substitute for the thorough and professional care of a licensed physician, psychologist, therapist, psychiatrist, addictionologist or addiction treatment facility.

TABLE OF CONTENTS

FOREWORD

By Angela Cornell, M.D.

I have been a practicing psychiatrist since 1980, after graduating from Emory University in Atlanta, Georgia and a Certified Addictionologist specializing in addiction medicine since 1992. Substance-addicted patients have come to me for help from all socioeconomic levels and all racial, ethnic and gender backgrounds. From the barely educated to Ivy League Ph.D.s, from day laborers to the most highly-regarded executives, my patients come from all walks of life. Yet all of them are confronted by the same roadblocks of ignorance and helplessness when they first try to face their addictions. Perhaps those patients for whom struggles with addiction and attempts to recover are hardest are healthcare professionals. For them, access to drugs, especially prescription drugs, is incredibly easy and they are often lulled into believing that their high levels of education and professional experience should protect them from temptation or prepare them to quit at the first sign of dependence.

Physicians, nurses, pharmacists, dentists and other healthcare professionals number among those most at risk for addiction to prescription medication. These professionals, like others who suffer from addiction, often try to explain away their drug abuse with excuses like: I was stressed/afraid/tired/overworked/in pain; my husband/partner/boss/children/parents expected too much from me and I couldn't meet their expectations; I couldn't relax; I didn't have time to think/I didn't think/I couldn't think. The difference between these professionals and those who do not work in the medical field is that healthcare professionals don't need to make doctor appointments, don't need to persuade first one doctor then another across town to write out prescriptions; they can simply wait until their colleagues look the other way.

It's easy. The irony is that despite being surrounded by other trained health-care professionals, these individuals feel as most people dependent on drugs do: absolutely alone, helpless and, yes, ignorant when the practice of self-medication evolves into a self-destructive habit.

It is in response to the needs of all persons addicted to prescription and over-the-counter medication that Cindy R. Mogil, a professional healthcare provider who struggled with her own addiction to prescription drugs, has founded Prescription Anonymous, the only self-help support group of its kind, in Atlanta, Georgia. Since 1998, this group has not only survived but thrived because of Cindy's diligence and dedication. She knows, as do I, how difficult it is to confront a group of strangers and confess not only one's difficulties, but one's need for education and support. For this reason, she has written this book, a lay person's guide to prescription and over-the-counter pill addiction. Cindy draws on her personal experience and the experiences of others who are fighting daily to recover from the mental, emotional and spiritual poverty that defines drug addiction. In this book, Cindy extends a much-needed invitation to all people who could be on the path to recovery if only someone would point the way. She's pointing the way. I, too, invite you to come along.

Angela Cornell, M.D.
November 20, 2000

ACKNOWLEDGMENTS

Among my many blessings was being led to Letitia Sweitzer. Her insightful editorial skills, generosity, vision and guidance made our collaboration a joy. Her devotion to this project and respect for my work is evident throughout this book; I will forever be grateful.

I especially would like to thank those who shared their personal stories of recovery. Though many have chosen to remain anonymous, I would like to thank in particular the following who were identified by first name only: Michael, Kevin, Pat, David, Shawna, Carol, Brandon and Tom.

I thank Dr. Angela Cornell, for her wisdom, compassion and ability to both pull me from the depths of despair and help me find the courage to embrace recovery without fear.

Special thanks to the following people who generously lent time and expertise thus making this book possible: Dr. Robert A. Schlampp, B.S., D.C., J. Bertram Solomon, Jr., B.S., D.C., Dianne McClintock Callahan, Floyd P. Garrett, M.D., Caroline Kerry Hirshfield, Benzodiazepine Anonymous, Nan H. Davis, R.Ph., M.S. and Pharmacists Anonymous.

A word of sincere thanks to my friends who have seen me through it all! Thank you for your encouragement, support and friendship: Angela Perkins, Betsy Hester, Cheryl Bean, Gloria Hunnicutt, Cheralee Rater, Michael Cartwright and Patch Adams.

Finally, I would like to express my appreciation to the many creative people working behind the scenes on my behalf: my agent, Thomas Fensch of New Century Literary Agency; New Horizon Press: Dr. Joan Dunphy, Rebecca Sheil, Lynda Hatch, Joseph Marron, JoAnne Thomas; cover designer, Robert Aulicino; photographer, Deborah Safaie @ Studio D.

INTRODUCTION
My Story

I am a prescription medication addict. The number of times I drove under the excessive influence of prescription drugs is too great to count. The ease with which I obtained Demerol injections from different clinics and emergency rooms is frightening. I'd drive home afterward knowing my mind was so impaired I could hurt or kill myself or someone else with my car. I had reached the point of no return and I wasn't sure I cared anymore. I felt alone, misunderstood, severely depressed and hopeless.

While driving home on the highway one day, something strange happened. Numbness besieged my face, neck and arms, paralyzing me with fear. Though I was only ten miles from home, at that moment I had no idea where I was. Confused and disoriented, I managed to call my husband on my cell phone to tell him I had taken a wrong turn and couldn't find my way back home. It was the first time I had ever told him I needed help for anything. Sitting in my car in the emergency lane, a shaking hand holding the cell phone to my ear, I could barely understand my husband's directions. Frightened and in tears, all I could think was, *How could this have happened to me?* I felt certain I could never reveal to my husband what was really going on. We had been together for nine years and he never suspected that I was anything but a well-adjusted, happy, normal adult. After all this time, how could I tell him that my "friends"—the prescription pills I abused to numb emotional pain—were now my predators?

When family and friends and even doctors first learn of a person's prescription medication addiction, they often ask incredulously, "How did you ever get into this mess?" They seem ready to accept that celebrities in big cities with their grow-up-too-fast, jet set lifestyles can easily fall prey to such problems, but a regular person like you? It couldn't happen to them, they think—you can hear it in their voices—so they can't imagine how it happened to you. Well, it can and does.

For some people, hereditary traits, environment and family structure interplay to create a susceptibility to addiction. One common precursor to addiction is emotional pain. For many people, emotional pain begins in early childhood. That's what happened to me. My emotional pain took root when I was only ten years old.

I had just turned ten when I was molested at an ice-skating rink. One night while playing tag with friends, I jumped over a high snow bank at the end of the ice rink to hide and avoid being tagged out of a game. A young man who had joined the game skated over to the bank after me where no one could see. As I lay there in the snow, he climbed over the bank and rolled right on top of me. Surprised and frightened by his sudden presence, I lay there in stunned silence. I tried to squirm my way out from under him, but he grabbed my arms so tightly I couldn't move. Then he began touching my chest. I tried to tell him to stop, but I couldn't get the words out. Almost as quickly as it started, he abruptly let me go, telling me to never reveal to anyone what happened or I would suffer the consequences. I pretended like nothing happened, afraid of what he might do to me if anyone found out. The next night, I reluctantly went back to the ice rink with my friends. Again, the young man caught me by surprise and the nightmarish event repeated itself. The next time I encountered him, he put his hand down my pants. I heard his breathing begin to labor and he moaned as he touched me. This time I could not keep quiet. I began to cry and in a small voice begged him to stop, but he refused. After what seemed like a lifetime, he took his hands off me and once again threatened to hurt me if I told a soul. I walked home in fear and shame as tears flowed down my cheeks in the cold, windy night. Thankfully, I never saw him again, but the effect he had on my life was profound.

I never told my parents about the young man or what he had done to me because I thought they would be angry. I didn't want to be scolded or told that it was my fault. I was afraid my family would make me feel worse about myself than I already did. Over the next three years I survived life and my parents' divorce by withdrawing from the world and becoming extremely shy, sensitive and insecure in the process.

One day, a classmate approached me and handed me a little blue pill. She told me she could see I was often sad and the pill would make my world a better and happier place to live in. I couldn't wait to take this "happy pill." I found out later that the pill was called "speed" (an amphetamine). When I took the pill, I felt carefree, rid of all my uncomfortable emotions and feelings. I liked feeling that way. Through that drug, I had found a place to which I could escape from my fears and loneliness. I was fourteen and a freshman in high school. I continued using speed regularly until my junior year in high school. One day my mother approached me, saying she suspected I was on drugs. I felt so guilty and ashamed for disappointing her that I abruptly stopped taking my "happy pill." She never asked why I had taken the pills and I certainly never volunteered any information about my emotional state.

Ten days after my eighteenth birthday, I was driving my car on my way to pick up a girlfriend to enjoy a night of dancing. To my surprise and shock, a pedestrian came darting out into the street seemingly unconcerned about the busy oncoming traffic. As the man came to a stop in my lane, I realized in that split second that he didn't appear to have any plans to get out of the street nor would I have time to avoid colliding with him. My heart pounded as I slammed on the brakes as hard as I could, silently praying for a miracle to avoid a terrible accident. My worst fears were realized when suddenly, I saw a slim body collide with my left fender then roll across the hood as the car skidded sideways. I remember the frightened look on his face as he rolled off my hood and landed face down on the sidewalk. Despite my own shock, I immediately sprang into action. Jumping out of my car, I screamed out for someone to call for an ambulance. When I reached the young man's body, I ripped off my jacket and gently placed it under his head. The young man died three days later of massive internal and brain injuries. He was twenty-one years old. His name was Andrew.

Even though I was found to not be at fault for the accident, the tragedy caused me to again isolate myself from my family and friends. I couldn't sleep, eat or talk to anyone. Seeing my despondency, my mother became fearful that I might try to commit suicide. She turned to my father for help and they decided it would be best for me to live with him. I was so distraught I wasn't able to make any decisions for myself, so I went along with whatever they suggested. Counseling was never an option approved of by my mother or father. They both felt I didn't need outside help from anyone and could heal myself. To them, this was just a car accident and I needed to move on with my life. But I just couldn't. I couldn't even look at myself in the mirror and I didn't know how much more guilt I could endure. I wasn't even sure I would be missed if I died. Isolation, devastation and severe depression took over my life for the next five years.

My stepmother, however, saw how much pain I was in and suggested that I might seek help through counseling to talk out my feelings. This would be my first encounter with therapy. I didn't have a clue how I could talk to a stranger, but it was a chance I needed to take. My life depended on it.

The County Health Department therapist walked in, introduced himself and blurted out, "So why are you here?" As I nervously stared at the floor, I gave him a short story of my past, not fully understanding how to respond to such a broad question. When my forty-five minutes were up, he said to me in an insensitive tone, "You need to forget about your accident. You said it yourself: It wasn't your fault. If you keep telling yourself you can't forget, then you never will go on with your life. Here, try some Valium. It should help."

Without hesitation, I started taking Valium along with high doses of sleeping pills he also prescribed. I felt lightheaded. I liked the sensation of carefree thoughts and the floating effects the drugs had over me. I didn't have fear, worry or depression. In fact, I didn't have any feelings anymore. I simply enjoyed the peace.

After a few weeks of what I felt was "useless therapy," I stopped making appointments. I knew what I needed to do to feel better: take enough pills to blot out the painful feelings and memories. I enjoyed numbness and didn't want to come back to reality, not for a while anyway. I was able to manipulate the receptionist at the counselor's office to refill my prescriptions about six times before I was told I needed to make another appointment.

The ease with which I could get prescriptions and refills from other healthcare providers surprised me. I decided I didn't need help from the county therapist or anyone else. I had made a new friend and it came in the form of a pill. It would be there when I needed it to be, any time, any place. To comfort, to calm, to numb. My world turned into manipulation and lies to family, friends and in the work place. Over the next fifteen years I manipulated doctors, dentists, therapists, emergency room personnel, pharmaceutical drug representatives and friends to get an array of different pills. Topping my list of choice pills were Librium, Darvon, Elavil, Demerol, Haldol, Halcion, Tranxene, Darvocet, Percocet, Percodan, Flexeril, Xanax and Ativan, to name a few. The healthcare providers I manipulated were prescribing medications based on the symptoms I told them, with an accompanying performance that would usually convince them they were doing the right thing. As my tolerance to pills grew so did the number of pills I took daily, sometimes up to fifteen or more a day. I started taking my pills the minute I woke up, with no preference to what kind of pill I took. I had pills for breakfast, lunch and dinner. I took a few more pills for sleep. I replaced food with pills and eventually mixed them with alcohol to speed up the effects. My weight dropped from 124 to 104 pounds within six weeks and I still didn't think anything was wrong.

I perhaps reached my lowest point while working at a cardiology office after eighteen years of experience in the healthcare profession. One day the doctor asked me to prep a patient for a Treadmill Stress Test. We used the treadmill to monitor the patient's heart rate at different speeds while he walked on the moving platform. As the treadmill's speed was increased, the patient became short of breath and began experiencing chest pain. The cardiologist ordered me to stop the treadmill immediately. Because I was high on pills, however, I couldn't locate the stop switch quickly enough and the patient fell off the platform. Fortunately, the cardiologist was able to catch the man so he didn't fall to the floor. The patient was shaken, but luckily was not hurt during the ordeal. I couldn't explain my behavior—my failure—to the cardiologist or to the patient, let alone forgive myself for my actions. That day I knew I had a real problem.

I found a new therapist who, realizing I was in danger of committing suicide, saw me the same day. She admitted me into the hospital for drug overdose, anxiety and severe depression. I was evaluated and put on a suicide watch while detoxing off pills and alcohol. I was in the treatment facility for ten days. I still denied that I had a serious problem. Nevertheless, I adhered to their rules. Finally, on the eleventh day, I was released.

Relapse came quickly. Within two months I was back to my old habits, manipulating doctors any way I could to maintain my supply of pills. One day, I noticed tingling in my arms and numbness in my jaw. I called my therapist to tell her. Again, fearing I had overdosed and might be contemplating suicide, she told me to return to the hospital. I refused to go. However, without my knowing it, she dialed 911 and called for an emergency paramedic to come to my house. I had previously mentioned to her that we had a gun in the house, so she told the emergency medical services I might be armed and dangerous. While I still talked with her on the phone, the doorbell rang. I put the phone down and answered the door. There stood three police officers with their guns drawn asking, "Do you have a weapon in your hands?" I said no and held up my empty hands as proof. They took me back to the treatment facility, where I finally admitted I was powerless over my addiction and needed help. I wasn't in denial any longer.

Withdrawal, however, does not make a pretty story. My discomfort ranged from physical pain—headaches and muscle aches—to emotional pain—wild mood swings, the strong urge to use drugs again and suicidal thoughts. And withdrawal doesn't mean just getting off the drug, giving up the "high" or pleasurable feelings. It also means facing life. When I was on drugs, I was able to mask my problems and hide from reality. Once I was off drugs, the problems were still there waiting for me. Now I had to deal with all the hurt that made me turn to drugs in the first place. Feeling pain meant I was returning to reality again and it was a frightening place in which to be. To be vulnerable to other people after being shielded for years from whatever personal pain I had to face was hard. Then on top of that pain, I was now afraid of being judged harshly as a recovering addict. If I had had the strength for all this, I wouldn't have been on pills in the first place! I had to decide if I wanted to live more than I wanted to die. I had to find self-respect and to love myself. If I couldn't find purpose and goals for myself, it would be hard not to relapse. If I didn't love myself, then pills would always be predators waiting for me to experience a moment of weakness.

Over the first two weeks of my hospitalization, I listened and shared stories in both individual and group therapy. For the first time in years, I felt hopeful.

Admitting I was powerless over any mood-altering substance was my first step to recovery. The second was to find a therapist who could help me move on with my life. The third was to find a sponsor who could give me guidance and support during recovery.

Since then, I have learned how to keep promises to myself and to always be truthful, honest and open-minded. I will always be an addict, meaning I will always be tempted. But now I understand I have choices in life and I must use those choices wisely. These insights have come to me the hard way. I can only keep these gifts that I have gained through recovery by sharing them with others. That is the reason I founded Prescription Anonymous, a recovery group for people like me, and the reason I wrote this book.

ADDICTION:
"How did I get into this mess?"

All of the people who have joined Prescription Anonymous, the group I founded, have distinct yet disquietingly similar stories about how and why they became addicted to prescription and/or over-the-counter drugs.

Kevin is a salesman and his story, like mine, illustrates a decades-long addiction rising out of a need to escape some lasting childhood hurt.

Kevin's Story

I was a very shy and insecure child by the age of three or four. Something happened at that age between my father, brother and me. I cannot recall the details, but I vividly remember the result. I sat on the couch in our living room and thought, "I will never let myself get close to anyone, because I will be hurt." And I didn't.

By the time I reached fifteen years old, I had begun to experiment with street drugs. With them, I found a way of covering up my fear of being close to people. By retreating into my fantasy world, I would not worry about other people at all. I drank sporadically, but developed an affinity for marijuana. I was playing "Russian roulette" with my own life, not thinking about the consequences. I loved the senseless feeling of being high. At twenty-one, I broke into a liquor store while I was away at college. I was arrested and charged with a felony. My parents, however, paid for a good lawyer who got me off with just probation. I remember wondering, Since there are no consequences for my actions, what else can I get away with?

All through my twenties I abused painkillers and depressants, including over-the-counter medicines, just to get high. They were cheaper than street drugs and they were legal. But after I'd quickly built up a tolerance to these, I needed stronger and higher doses of medication. I stole pills from my friends' parents' medicine cabinets while they were home, even broke into my friends' homes to steal pills while they were gone. My conscience never bothered me; it never once told me this was wrong! I was in control or so I thought.

I took all kinds of pills, drank liquor, smoked pot, sometimes all at the same time, without thinking about what I was doing to myself. I had developed a habit and didn't know I would have to confront my demons one day. I frequently got sick from pill and alcohol poisoning until I passed out. My body was physically wearing out and shutting down. It was a miracle that I didn't die from all the binges. Depression developed, but I still somehow managed to put on a performance of being focused and normal while at work or with friends and family. My friends who saw me drink never voiced their concerns over my consumption or they just chose not to say anything. And it quickly became apparent that very few people get concerned if they see you putting a pill in your mouth!

Through manipulation and lies, I persuaded my dentist to write painkiller prescriptions for fake toothaches. I never paid any attention to the instructions from my dentist or the ones that came with the medicine. I often consumed twice the amount prescribed.

My life was empty. Isolation and depression ruled me. I kept to myself outside of work and home. Most of my hours were dedicated to getting high, alone. I remember thinking, What a waste! *But I couldn't stop and I didn't know how to ask for help.*

I met my wife when I was thirty-eight years old. We were like two peas in a pod. We both enjoyed drinking and partying, although her drinking was not as chronic as mine was. After we were married, the pressures of marriage, home ownership and being a stepfather began to weigh heavily on me. At forty-one, I changed jobs and we moved closer to my work. We also had a son of our own by this time. With so many mounting pressures, my anxiety became uncontrollable. I was illegally taking prescription painkillers now, but my wife never suspected that I might be addicted to pills. If she had suspected, she would have done something about it, but I had her convinced that I was all right.

Once I went to my dentist with a legitimate problem for which he gave me painkillers. These ran out after a few days, so I had to get "creative." I returned to him and lied about the severity of my toothache from a root canal he had done. After a month, he would no longer give me any more pills or refills, so I went to my wife's dentist, who, for a while, became my "Dr. Feelgood." If I asked for painkillers, he would prescribe them without question or hesitation. Over the course of three months, he wrote between fifteen to twenty prescriptions for Percodan.

One day, even "Dr. Feelgood" refused to write any more prescriptions, so again I got "creative" and decided to write my own prescription. I took the prescription that the dentist had written for me, copied it, used Wite Out to cover up the old prescription and then wrote out new prescriptions. I never felt guilty and I never thought about the consequences that I would have to pay if I ever got caught. I never had to pay consequences before, why should I pay for this?

After twenty-five forged prescriptions, I got caught! While I was at work one day, a detective went to my house and spoke with my wife. She was stunned and could only listen in shock and amazement when the detective pulled out all the forged prescriptions to show her. He was a kind man, because he did not issue a warrant for my arrest, but only told her he needed to talk with me.

My wife called me at the office and made up a story to get me home, fearing I might run from this problem if I knew what was happening. I'll never forget the shame I felt when my wife confronted me at home. In tears and anger, she asked, "How could you do this to us and this family?" For the first time, I was overwhelmed with fear and remorse. I realized I was inflicting the same hurt I suffered as an abused child on those who loved me.

I obtained a lawyer and he was able to talk the detective out of arresting me. He "took care of it"—familiar words to me, the same ones used when I was arrested as a teen. As a result of this crisis, I tried Alcoholics Anonymous for the first time, but I felt I was wasting my time, listening to everybody pouring out their stories of sorrow and grief. One week of meetings was all I could stand.

Soon I was going to dentists again, lying about tooth pain to get yet another supply of painkillers. I did this for a few months until my wife caught me with some pills. She threatened to leave me if I didn't get help. I tried Alcoholics Anonymous again, for her, not for myself. Within a couple of weeks I was forging prescriptions again with no end in sight. I was in a nightmare and couldn't wake myself up.

When I could no longer find a doctor to write prescriptions for me, I used fake names and new pharmacies to get my forged prescriptions filled. After three months of this insanity, I exhausted myself and could not go on.

*I was killing myself, a slow death, and for the first time I was afraid of
dying. I returned to my old therapist, admitted what I had done and asked
for help. There had to be a better way of life for me, because my way was
destroying all I loved, my family and myself.*

*Somehow I got the strength to tell my wife the truth of what I had done.
Thankfully, she decided to stay with me. I have accepted the fact that I have
a disease called prescription addiction as well as alcoholism and that my
recovery requires a commitment from me and from my family.*

*I feel differently about recovery this time. Admitting my wrongs and
making amends was my first step. I now have a sponsor, who I talk to every
day, who gives me guidance.*

*I attend meetings every week at Prescription Anonymous and
Alcoholics Anonymous to get the support and understanding I so desperately need. I learned that thousands of people die from this disease every
year. I'm so grateful I found help in time and pray that others find help and
support somewhere before it's too late.*

In addition to ameliorating emotional pain, another common precursor to
addiction is the legitimate prescription of drugs for physical pain. Painkillers
and other medications affect different people in different ways. While some
patients can take a drug briefly and be glad for the physical relief it brings without experiencing any unusual alteration of mood, others may experience
euphoria, which they find they love and do not want to give up. When misused
by the patient and/or prescribed too freely by the physician, an appropriate
drug becomes a trap that enmeshes the patient in a lifetime of torment.

Shawna is a recovered prescription addict who has a story that unfolds
in several places throughout this book.

Shawna's Story

*At the ripe old age of five, I underwent open-heart surgery. The surgery
was successful, but what changed my life more than the surgery itself was
the little pill the doctor gave me afterward for pain. I have forgotten the
pain, but I remember the pills. They gave me a wonderful, oh-so-happy feeling I had never felt before, could not have imagined before. And I did not
want to give them up.*

*"Mommy, it hurts so bad!" I don't know how many times I uttered these
words as a child. I remember there was a small merry-go-round outside on
the floor of the children's ward. I begged my father to take me there one
sunny afternoon. I asked him to push me faster and faster. Then I faked a*

pain in my chest. I knew that if I said I was hurting, they would give me some "stuff" to make me feel all nice and warm. Nurses and doctors came running. I can vividly picture my father's face as they listened for chest sounds. He was devastated, tears rolling down his cheeks, thinking he was the cause of my pain. That was the beginning of a way of life, full of deceit, which still haunts me today.

As a young girl of ten, I was diagnosed with scoliosis, a curvature of the spine. The doctors took a "wait and see" approach for a couple of years, but it progressively got worse. Finally, I was fitted for a Milwaukee back brace. It was made of steel and hard plastic and enclosed my entire torso and spine. I hated it for making me so unattractive and a target for teasing. Thus, I was pleased beyond delight when two years later the orthopedic surgeon said that he needed to do surgery. I was thirteen. Little did I know just how excruciating spinal surgery would be. I remember it hurt to even move my fingers, my toes or my mouth. I was in so much pain that I prayed to die. Several times I screamed until someone gave me morphine. Three days after my back surgery, my stomach began to bloat to the point that I looked nine months pregnant. I was only one hundred pounds. They would come in and push on it, asking me if it hurt. Even though it genuinely hurt, I would cry out in a much more dramatic way than was warranted. I was once again rushed into surgery. They were sure it was appendicitis. When they opened me up, they found my appendix to be in marvelous shape. So they kept cutting deeper and wider only to find an ovarian cyst the size of a grapefruit. They removed it and stitched me back up—the scar ended up spanning the entire stomach region. Not only was I recovering from spinal surgery, now I had to deal with staples all down my front. The doctors, knowing this, kept me completely doped up for a good month. Then they sent me home with enough narcotics to last a couple of months. I took them all.

I remember thinking at some point that I probably didn't need to keep taking the drugs, but since the doctor prescribed them, I should. My parents were always after me, "Shawna, do what the doctor says!" I had no idea that the pills were addictive. I didn't even know what addiction was. My father should have. He was in law enforcement, with special training in narcotics investigation. But I was his little girl who could do no wrong. If I was in pain, he was going to make sure that I was taken care of. Who would've guessed that his "angel girl" would end up being a hard-core prescription drug addict?

When the drugs were gone, I was in a world of hurt—psychologically. I couldn't function. My mother would tell me to "quit moping around...and stand up straight!" I was in a black hole that I couldn't seem to get out of. I couldn't understand why. Why wasn't I like my six brothers and sisters? Why couldn't I be carefree like my schoolmates? I quickly learned to put on a face of confidence and radiance. I knew what my parents and teachers wanted, so I gave it to them. I didn't want anyone to see my gut-wrenching depression and low self-worth. So I excelled for them. I performed regularly, winning awards for musical talent. I was the lead in school musicals and the solo voice in many choirs. I loved the art of drama, because I could literally get out of myself for a while and become an entirely different person. But in between productions, I would break down. I needed to be in that warm place again where I didn't have to think about anything.

During this time, I recalled what the doctor said after my last surgery, "Teenage girls get cysts all the time. But for some reason it's more painful for some. It looks like your daughter may be in this category. You'll want to keep an eye on her ten to fourteen days after her periods each month." That was a green light to me. I kept track of my period and, fourteen days to the day, I would feign horrible abdominal pain. My parents would rush me to the gynecologist, who would do a pelvic exam. Ninety percent of the time they would go in surgically and remove a small cyst. This meant weeks of painkillers. Sometimes my doctor would ask me to ride out the pain and call in a prescription for sixty Vicodin. This was fine by me. By the time I was eighteen, I had endured approximately twenty unnecessary surgeries. I felt truly evil for being so deceitful.

Not everyone who becomes addicted to prescription drugs—or any substance—acquires the addiction as early as Kevin, Shawna and I did. Not all abusers have suffered from childhood traumas or physical pain.

The next story comes from Pat, who first fell under the spell of drugs in middle age.

Pat's Story

I didn't become addicted to any substance until I was over fifty. I didn't even like the floaty feeling my first prescription pills gave me. But I was, I now realize, addicted to power—the power I had over my husband as a caregiver. For twenty-seven years, I was married to an alcoholic who leaned on me to take care of everything, including the bills and paying for tickets he acquired while driving under the influence of alcohol. I even made the important decisions in our lives, whether it was buying major appliances or deciding on the best schools for our children. This gave me tremendous power in the marriage. I liked the feeling of that power, the adrenaline high

I felt over someone else even when he turned from Dr. Jekyll to Mr. Hyde from drinking. When he decided to seek help through Alcoholics Anonymous, I was glad that he was trying to control his drinking, but fearful for myself, because I knew I would lose my control over him and our lives would be changed.

He had an affair with someone he met at Alcoholics Anonymous and decided to leave our marriage for her. I felt relieved that I wouldn't be living with an alcoholic any more, but in losing my power, I was scared and alone for the first time in twenty-seven years.

A few months after the divorce, I went to see our family doctor, complaining of anxiety, depression and tension headaches. She gave me a prescription for a hundred tablets of Fiorinal No. 3, a pain medication for the headaches. She never warned me of the addictive tendencies of the drug nor did she instruct me on how to take them. She even gave me three refills!

Even though I didn't like them at first, after a few weeks, I came to love the little pills. I would count out my feel-good pills in the morning to make sure I had a full day's supply. I would have never dreamed that pills could become such a powerful part of my life. I not only had lost control over my ex-husband, but now I had lost control of myself. I no longer took my medication for pain, but for coping. They made my stressful day more bearable. They gave me a second wind. They made me excel or so I thought.

I really thought I was on top of it all, staying in touch with reality. I was blind to the multitude of compulsive behaviors in my life, like shopping, overeating and hiding in seclusion. Once my tolerance to the pills developed, it was virtually impossible for my friends or family to accurately gauge the extent of my dependence. I could appear completely normal during an extended part of my day.

Subconsciously, I guess I knew I was harming my body. It started with my kidneys. I saw blood in my urine and had numerous kidney infections. My doctor did all the tests and I ended up going to a kidney specialist who put me on a medication called Macrodantin to clear up the infection. I looked the medication up in my Physicians Desk Reference *which stated that Macrodantin could lessen the effects of Fiorinal. I decided not to take it, even if it meant further damaging my kidneys. Nothing was going to lessen the effects of my feel-good pill, no matter what. I had to have my Fiorinal every day.*

One Friday I realized I didn't have enough pills to last through the weekend, so I decided to call in sick at work and made an emergency doctor visit. I perfected my "performance" in my car and in the waiting room,

visualizing exactly what I'd say and how I would act to get my fix of pills.
I even wore sloppy clothes, no make-up and messy hair to look the part of
a person in pain. It worked well. Too well.

Back at home, high under the influence of the pills, I had an accident. I
stumbled into a tall piece of furniture and a one-hundred-pound metal light
fixture fell on my head causing a severe head injury. I managed to get to
the phone to call 911. I needed surgery to stop internal bleeding inside my
head. It was while I was recuperating in the hospital that I had to face up
to my addiction.

After two days of not having any Fiorinal, I began to feel nervous and
soon my anxiety returned with a vengeance—classic signs of withdrawal.
Because of my severe injuries, I was refused my Fiorinal, which I had
brought with me to the hospital. I was told that because of the other med-
ications they were giving me, Fiorinal would hinder my treatment for
internal bleeding. My withdrawal symptoms were becoming more notice-
able to the nurses and my doctor. They suspected that I might be addicted
to a substance.

I was ashamed and embarrassed about having to ask for help, but I
had no choice. I was powerless and I had to admit it to someone. At first,
my doctor did not understand how or why I had gotten myself addicted to
Fiorinal. It was difficult to be truthful with him, but ever since the day I
finally explained to him about my addiction, he has been a source of com-
fort, empathy, guidance and support. He has directed me to people who
could help me through my recovery.

I received my initial treatment through Chemical Dependency
Services. This organization gave me the steps to recovery and offered sup-
port groups where I could talk freely about the anger and frustration I felt
about my divorce. I've also learned about the co-dependency I practiced
throughout my marriage. I am learning how to take care of myself for the
first time in my life.

I once viewed alcoholics as having weak character; I had no sympathy
for them. Now I know I was no better than my alcoholic husband. I am as
sick as he was. Alcohol was just not my "drug of choice." I now understand,
after all these years, the misery and pain my husband must have gone
through.

I'll admit that some days I still try to talk myself into believing that my
addiction was not really that bad. Denial pops into my still vulnerable mind.
It has taken time for me to "wake up" and see how much of life I was missing.
The deeper I get involved with real life, the less power my addiction has.

Recovery is a journey on new paths every day. I have found myself wanting to try them all, but, knowing I must be careful not to get lost along the way, I have finally found that right path. I would gladly share it with others. I call it freedom.

Now that Kevin, Shawna, Pat and I have told you how we got into the mess of prescription addiction, here is what the experts say about us and millions of others in the same boat. First of all, even though we may have been given our first addictive medication by someone else, perhaps medical professionals and perhaps for legitimate reasons, very soon we misused or abused the substance. The definition of medication abuse is the use of any prescription medication not specifically prescribed for you or the use of a prescription or over-the-counter medication in any way that is different from the instructions given by the doctor or printed on the label of the medication.

The most addictive medications, whether prescription or over-the-counter medication, fall into three categories: stimulants, narcotics and sedatives. Scientific research has shown that when these addictive or abusable drugs bombard the system, they change the biochemistry of the brain. In this way, drugs themselves cause addiction when they are taken often enough, for long enough and in sufficient quantities. Some individuals are much more vulnerable to addiction than others, as with any disease, but even the less vulnerable can become physically addicted through use and misuse.

Steven E. Hyman, M.D., director of the National Institute for Mental Health, explains it this way: "After ongoing infiltration over time, drugs insidiously shift the brain's circuitry until they have eventually usurped control of the brain's normal mechanism for regulating behavior."[1]

Dr. Hyman likens addictive drugs to Trojan horses. In masquerade they enter the brain, but, as they wreak havoc with the brain's natural mechanism of regulating pleasure, the apparent gift becomes an agent of betrayal.

These drugs initially fool the brain into producing extra dopamine. Dopamine is the major chemical substance or neurotransmitter in the brain's normal reward circuit. The release of extra dopamine induces feelings of well-being or euphoria. Whereas short-term use of some prescription drugs increases dopamine levels, the brain, which tries to keep the body's chemicals in balance, physically adapts to chronic use by actually decreasing dopamine levels as well as the ability to produce it.

For the prescription addict, abuse often begins the moment a pharmacist fills a doctor's prescription. Instead of taking the medicine as prescribed, the abuser soon increases the amount and frequency without the doctor's knowledge or approval in order to get more of the desired effect. As the abuse becomes more frequent, depleted levels of dopamine result in both depression and craving—important elements of addiction and the key factors leading to relapse. This is how addiction happens and, as you can see, it is both physiological and psychological.

Floyd P. Garrett, M.D., complains of confusing terminology. He calls the physical addiction that Dr. Hyman describes "physical dependence." He contrasts this to "psychological dependence," a phrase that describes a dependence on something that is not necessarily physically powerful, on a placebo or sugar pill, for example. A person is psychologically dependent on something because he feels better with it in spite of no pharmacological changes. One could be psychologically dependent on a substance, on an activity such as thumb sucking or on a lucky charm. Sometimes a psychological dependence is relatively harmless except that giving it up is problematic. The term "addiction" Dr. Garrett reserves for that complex pattern of behavior characterized by "obsession with obtaining and using the drug, excessive, prolonged and harmful use despite adverse consequences and the mental defense mechanisms of denial, rationalization, minimization and justification."[2] While many people beat dependencies by a period of abstinence or a gradual withdrawal, those who are vulnerable become addicted.

And who are the vulnerable? The vulnerable may be those individuals whose lives include emotional suffering as in the first story in this chapter. We must not discount, however, individual differences in physical reaction. Different drugs affect different people in different ways. Appropriate dosages are not always predictable. Who knows which people will be sensitive to which drug? I have talked to people who have undergone surgery, taken the pain pills afterwards, were grateful for the relief from pain, but say that they didn't alter their mood at all. "Percocet did nothing for me," I've been amazed to hear people say. Percocet did everything for me; that's why I took more and more.

Here's a well-expressed insight shared by one recovering addict:

So many of us started taking the pills just to get a break from the pain. I don't know about you, but I never expected the sense of euphoria that comes along with it. I absolutely live for the first two hours after my pill kicks in. Sad thing is, I told my doctor this, too, and all he asked me is: would you prefer the pain? I honestly don't know anymore.

The addict is propelled from his first flirtation with misuse into a pattern of addiction and denial that leads to self-destruction. "The dangers posed by prescription drugs are not all obvious," says Donald Healy, program manager for a recovery clinic in Detroit. "As users start taking larger doses, their tolerance to the drugs' effects increases, but the lethal limit does not. You're still functioning, walking and talking on doses that would have knocked out a normal person, all the while inching closer to a dose that can kill you without warning," Healy explains.[3]

Prescription and over-the-counter medication abuse or misuse can hook anyone. The abuse of legal drugs occurs in a variety of ways, in all segments of our population, in all kinds of neighborhoods and workplaces. What level of abuse will have an addictive effect on you depends on your physical and emotional vulnerability to addiction. The lucky ones get away without addiction. But how many are unlucky?

Almost nine million people annually abuse or become addicted to prescription drugs, according to the 1999 National Household Survey on Drug Abuse.[4] Two million of those addicted become seriously ill and 125,000 **die** every year. The common, immediate causes of death are liver or kidney failure, heart rhythm problems and bone marrow destruction.

Until recently, law enforcement, healthcare professionals and the general public have placed little emphasis on this huge problem of illegal misuse of prescription drugs. Prosecutors say that the way the laws are written in most states allows healthcare professionals to escape serious drug trafficking charges if they have written prescriptions, no matter how fraudulent. In fact, in 1994 in California, 75 percent of physicians convicted of prescription drug crimes kept their licenses.

In one regional report, prescription drug-related crimes included:

A woman treated at a clinic who had been charged by police with feeding her addiction to Vicodin by forging prescriptions;

A healthcare professional charged with stealing sample medications while at work and calling in prescriptions to pharmacies to obtain her own medication;

An ambulance driver charged with stealing painkillers while on the job from the patients he was transporting;

A social worker caught stealing pain medication from a cancer patient, telling police that no one would ever notice if one of the bottles went missing;

A mother charged with neglect after officials found out she was filling prescriptions for her sick child only to feed her own addiction and never giving the medication to her child.

"Sometimes, family members become actively involved in their loved ones' prescription drug abuse," says Frank Poloucek, Doctor of Pharmacy at the University of Illinois, Chicago. Family members give prescription drugs to their kids to calm them down or dope up their elderly relatives to keep them quiet. Poloucek calls such abuse "assault with a chemical weapon."[5] Moreover, healthcare professionals such as physicians and nurses, studies show, are addicted to prescription drugs at about the same rate as the general public.

The exact frequency of prescription drug abuse is unknown in the United States, but, according the United States Drug Enforcement Agency (DEA), prescription medications account for more than half of the twenty controlled substances most often involved in overdoses and other drug-related emergencies. Statistics supplied by the DEA indicate that more than 69,000 hospital emergency room visits involved the abuse of benzodiazepines, a category of prescription tranquilizers used to treat anxiety, stress and insomnia. Hospital emergencies involving the abuse of prescription medications in 1994 numbered more than 100,000, while in the same year approximately 63,000 emergency room visits were attributed to heroin addiction.

The abuse of prescription drugs is a particularly complex facet of America's drug problem, because, unlike illegal drugs, convenient access to prescription drugs must be maintained for legitimate purposes. Prescription drug abuse is often overlooked because people think that, if a doctor prescribes the drug and a pharmacist dispenses the medication, it can't be abused. It is difficult for most people to understand that prescription drugs can be every bit as addictive, destructive and craved as illicit drugs. I hope our stories have made this danger clear and helped readers understand how even ordinary people can fall into the trap of prescription addiction.

This chapter is intended to answer the question, "How did you ever get into this mess?" However, in order to give hope to all readers—those who are addicted, the families and friends of the addicted and the professional helpers—I want to remind you that the storytellers went on to eventual recovery. There is real hope glimmering at the end of even the most difficult stages of the journey to recovery, as you will see. Statistically, a full 50 percent of those who decide to beat addiction succeed. I hope reading this book will help you or someone you care about join the ranks of those fortunate individuals who have conquered their addictions.

DENIAL:

"I don't have a problem. I'm in control."

My husband and son used to watch me in disbelief and say, "Aren't you supposed to be taking only two of those pills?" This became a game of open-ended questions with a simple answer, "Oh, I have a higher than normal tolerance with this medication." They trusted me to tell the truth and didn't question me any further. I was home free, again.

Denial is a game we addicts play with our family, friends and associates. It is also a game we play by ourselves, like solitaire. We can play either functional or dysfunctional denial.

Functional denial occurs when you have convinced yourself that you know what's best for you, because you can still function normally. You feel you are actually being more productive on the job or at home with pills than without. You have completely resolved in your mind that it is all right to take more pills than directed without consequences. You keep this to yourself so others won't ask questions. You feel that as long as you aren't slurring your speech, stumbling over the furniture or falling down on the floor, you are still in control. You deny that drugs are in control.

Dysfunctional denial occurs when you have difficulty waking up or when you get up with a foggy mind in the morning, swallow stimulant pills before showering then try to converse with your loved ones, not paying attention or caring about what they have to say. Despite all this, you think you are okay. Dysfunctional denial means barely remembering driving under the influence of pills. If you didn't kill anyone, this was a good day!

Dysfunctional denial means loss of control of your life. It can include loss of a job, divorce or separation and isolation from friends. Days of happiness, a clear mind and genuine caring for someone else besides yourself are now gone. Despite this, you continue to tell yourself and others you don't have a problem.

Whether functional or dysfunctional, denial has several levels. Some level of denial occurs even in healthy people. Most of us have trouble admitting that a problem we don't want to deal with exists or we make excuses for what we know is our contribution to a problem. Healthy people deny up to a point; addicts deny way beyond health and reason. For addicts, it seems to make sense to protect the one thing that has long been a constant in our lives—pills.

At one level, we flat out deny our misuse of prescription drugs. Have you heard yourself say any of the following lines, which you now know to be untrue?

> I'm not addicted to my prescription drugs or over-the-counter medicines.
> I'm not misusing or abusing prescription drugs or over-the-counter medicines.
> I can stop taking this medication any time I choose.
> I don't try to hide any of my prescriptions or medications from family or friends.
> I take medicines as directed.
> I never mix mood-altering prescriptions with alcohol.
> I can function normally at home and work without mishap.

At another level of denial, addicts may not bother to hide their abnormal behaviors or symptoms, because they don't recognize these signs as being unusual. For example, I used to go up to girl friends and ask them for a pill or two from their prescriptions as casually as some people bum cigarettes. I didn't realize that I was doing anything out of the ordinary. If an addicted person's behavior has never gotten him or her arrested, then it must be acceptable, the reasoning goes. Such individuals are like speeders who say, "I don't speed" when they mean, "I have never gotten a ticket." And if a doctor hasn't identified their symptoms as dangerous, they're okay, right?

The emotional signals of addiction, including mood swings, isolation, boredom, unexpressed resentment and hatred, chronic depression and dishonesty, are usually recognized by family members first and later by friends and co-workers, but rarely by the addict, who sees the negative emotions as just a normal part of a disappointing life. Physical symptoms of abuse are also frequently misinterpreted. The addict and even his doctors may see the physical symptoms, but not connect them to drug abuse. These symptoms include liver or heart failure, frequent and lingering injuries, slurred speech, blackouts, decreased sex drive and overall deterioration of physical and emotional health. Failure to connect these symptoms to prescription drug abuse may even get additional drugs prescribed, which further feed the addiction.

At still another level of denial, the addict is more conscious of the problem and so tries harder to hide it. At this level, misuse of prescription drugs requires "justification" or rationalization. The abuser of prescription drugs may say one of the following:

> Accidents can happen to anyone.
> I was so depressed, I only took an extra pill or two to calm down.
> I was more upset than usual. One more pill couldn't hurt.
> I still can't sleep...my over-the-counter medicine said take one or two pills at bedtime. What's wrong with one more?
> It's none of your business how many pills I take. I'm fine.
> I need to lose weight fast so I will still be attractive.
> Sample medications are free, so no one will miss a few.
> I can't bear the pain. I need an extra pain pill now. It's only an hour before the next dose is due.

Do any of these lines sound familiar? Justification comes so easy. I remember. If you feel you have to justify your use of medication, you are probably in denial.

Notice also that several of the rationalizations above describe a degree of discomfort as intolerable: "so depressed," "can't sleep," "more upset," and "I can't bear." Our minds can play such evil tricks on us! As prescription addicts, we will create or exaggerate a symptom in our minds in order to justify taking any type of mood-altering pill available in the house. Our sick minds will somehow tell us that the pain is worse than it really is in order to justify taking the pills. The deceit not only seems to justify the misuse of the drug, but the drug serves as a reward or reinforcement for the pain or discomfort so that subsequent pain or discomfort actually increases in frequency or intensity. This sets up the next exaggerated pain, which is not long in coming. For example, an addict who takes a pill because she can't sleep is rewarding herself for the sleeplessness and the next night may toss and turn to get the same problem in order to justify the same solution. For people who enjoy the feeling of an altered mind, taking pills conditions the person to experience the symptom that requires the pill.

Finally, some people addicted to prescription drugs do see their own pattern of abuse fairly clearly. In fact, they have strong feelings of remorse and guilt over their out-of-control behavior with prescription drugs and nearly destroying lives including their own. To ease these unpleasant feelings, they take more pills. It's the only remedy they have mastered. They don't have the courage to admit to others that they have a problem or to seek out help. In fact, lack of courage underlies all forms of denial.

To some extent, denial works for a while. Addicts have to be really desperate to see that something else works better.

At Prescription Anonymous support groups, members often recall the denial that earlier kept them from seeking help.

"The idea of getting caught or being accused of abusing my prescriptions or over-the-counter medicines never played a part in my everyday scenario," one person told our support group recently.

"The thought that one day I might need to face my 'problem,' if I had one, never crossed my mind," another admitted. "I would probably never seek outside intervention because I believed I was still in control."

Another member in recovery shared his thoughts and memories. "At first I wasn't abusing my medications because I was taking them as directed. But when money problems and stress from issues with my family, wife and kids became unbearable, I had such a strong compulsion to take extra pills for anxiety, something to stay calmer than what the usual dosage prescribed. I chose to take an extra three pills one day, then five, eight, ten and the cycle of misuse began. I justified my abuse to myself and did not tell anyone."

During a group meeting, a recently widowed woman sadly related, "I never recognized my denial until after I stopped abusing anxiety medication and sleeping pills. I used these drugs to help me sleep and cope after my husband died. I was allowed to receive as many refills as I wanted with just a little persuasion on my part. The doctors who prescribed the drugs never told me how addictive they are. They simply said I should take them as needed, so I ended up taking as much as I wanted as often as I wanted. It seemed okay at the time, because it was all legal, aboveboard and approved by my doctors." The distinction of legality and doctor approval is a typical aspect of denial in the prescription drug addict. It leads her to falsely believe her problem isn't really a problem. After all, she is not some junkie on a street corner or doing drugs in a back alley. Her drugs are legal. Her doctor gave them to her. Thus, how could she be a "drug addict"?

Another member shared how denial contributed to her struggle with prescription drug addiction. "Denial for me meant refusing to believe the truth no matter what someone else said. I could justify my behavior and addictive habit to anyone, including myself. I self-medicated when I needed to, stopped or slowed down as I pleased and thought this was fine. I refused to ask for help; I was too proud, very independent, strong headed and thought I could take care of myself. I didn't want anyone telling me how many pills I could take. Pills were like trophies to me; I didn't want anyone else touching them."

I, too, denied my drug abuse even after I was in therapy. I had been severely depressed for months and my therapist prescribed anti-depressant pills. I never told my therapist that I had been misusing my pills for weeks, because I didn't think that someone else knew best for me. It wasn't anybody else's business. Besides, I knew how much my body could tolerate.

Aside from spending time with others in support group meetings now that I have conquered my addiction, I frequent Internet chat rooms devoted to discussing medication addiction. For many of the faceless, often anonymous, chat room members, this forum is the first place they go to admit they have drug problems. Others are in recovery and working to stay clean. Through the shared stories of painful struggles with prescription addiction, one element is consistent throughout: denial. The expression of denial, past or present, shared in these virtual chat rooms sound similar to those heard in physical support group meetings. For example, one woman felt her addiction to pills didn't make her a drug addict because "I am a white, middle-class woman. I had a well-paying job, a family, a home. I wasn't some person on the street living in the gutter."

Another woman admitted to the group of Internet "chatters" that she was shocked when addiction caught up with her. Like all of us, she just never thought it could affect her. "My ex-husband had addiction problems. Not me. I always thought it could never happen to me."

Denial can be subtle. It may take a long time and a lot of soul-searching for a recovering addict to even identify some of his past actions as denial. One wealthy man admitted it was denial that led him to choose an insurance-covered detoxification program instead of a rapid detoxification program that was significantly faster. At the time, he blamed the choice on frugality, but has since realized he was really allowing himself several more months in which to abuse prescription drugs than he would have had if he had chosen the rapid program.

Though some expressions of denial seem pretty straightforward, others are more complex. One woman with whom I chatted on the Internet shared her story, which included multiple levels of denial.

"I used alcohol at one point, but I didn't really like it and drinking went against my beliefs so I stopped. Later, after I was diagnosed with migraine headaches, I began abusing the Demerol and Percocet prescribed to me. They made me feel good. I thought it was okay. After all, if it wasn't, why did my doctor give them to me?"

I immediately recognized the many levels of denial she was experiencing. First, she claimed it was against her beliefs to misuse alcohol, so she stopped. In reality, she didn't like alcohol anyway. Yet with prescription drugs, she didn't see the abuse as a problem. After all, they made her feel good; she liked them. When she finally did see she had a problem, she placed the responsibility squarely on the shoulders of her doctor.

An admission of addiction combined with denial of the effect addiction has on others is another very common form of destructive thinking. Patti, a thirty-year-old woman who told me how she takes up to twenty pills a day, knows she is addicted and wants to stop, but assured me, "My family does not suffer from my abuse. I take care of my kids and I work." All I could think upon hearing her words was that I'd like to talk to Patti's husband, children and co-workers to see what they have to say about her behavior and actions. I suspect her drug addiction has a huge impact on them, whether Patti wants to admit it or not. Furthermore, her young children may seem oblivious to the problem now, but if asked years from now, the long-term effects of their mother's addiction will likely be evident. Chances are very good that Patti's home and work environments are not as healthy and happy as she claims them to be.

Denial seems so obvious to outsiders and even to drug abusers once they've quit. When wrapped up in one's medication addiction, however, it is difficult to see or think clearly. Few realize they are in denial. Instead, the addict angrily dismisses responsibility for his actions and blame is placed on others. One of the easiest and most common targets for the prescription medication addict's blame is his doctor. Thomas, who was still very much in the grip of denial, shared his feelings with our chat group.

"I can't confront a doctor again, so I borrowed a prescription from a friend. Now it's almost gone. What am I going to do? I hold these doctors responsible. They give refill after refill until you are hooked. Why are doctors able to do this to people?"

Peter, who has yet to begin addiction recovery, agreed with Thomas, adding his own complaints about doctors.

"They don't seem to ever want to take any of the blame. They don't tell you when you get the pills to beware, that they are very addictive."

To some extent, both Thomas and Peter have legitimate complaints. Physicians do have the responsibility to fully explain to a patient not only possible side effects, but the potential for addiction of any drug they prescribe. Nonetheless, blaming others, whether they deserve it or not, is a dangerous form of denial because it diverts energy and attention from the addict's responsibility to move forward in recovery. It creates anger instead of hope. Someone else may be responsible for your addiction, but you are responsible for your recovery.

Anger at people who try to help an addict or obstruct his drug abuse often fuels denial. Yet it is a natural reaction for many to view those who try to help as villains. One young woman, Tiffany, told the group about her pharmacist's attempt to intervene. At the time, his actions made Tiffany furious.

"I submitted a prescription from a doctor who wasn't my regular family doctor. My pharmacist caught it immediately. I think he suspected I was an addict already. He pulled me over to the side of the counter and told me how dangerous and addictive these drugs are. Then he suggested that I was an addict. I became irate."

Like all of us who have suffered with prescription addiction, Tiffany was at a point when she wasn't ready to face her problem. And she certainly wasn't pleased to have someone else point it out to her. Happily, she finally got help and came to realize the pharmacist did what he did because he really cared about her well-being and, in fact, may have saved her life. She was so touched by his kindness and concern that she has since gone back to tell him of her recovery and thank him for his compassion.

Another kind of denial involves obstructive thoughts. I call this "but I can't" denial. I have great sympathy for the "but I can'ts" because the basis of their reasoning is real. They say, "I know I'm addicted, I know it's ruining my life, but I can't go into treatment because...." The lists of reasons that follow usually sound legitimate. Whether they are financial constraints or childcare issues, they are real concerns that take priority over recovery for many people. Here are some examples of the "but I can'ts" I've been told throughout the years:

"My new doctor gave out narcotics freely until I mentioned to her that I felt addicted. Then she cut me off and told me I needed to detox. I cannot go into detox because I have three kids in school."

"My wife stays at home with the kids and I am the one who works outside the home. If I leave for treatment, then she and the kids will lose everything. I can't lose my job."

An even more prevalent reason than financial burdens or time constraints for many who use the "but I can't" excuse is the fear of public exposure. I have seen that fear expressed over and over in support group meetings and during Internet chat room discussions:

"I would really like to stop, but I live in a small town and am too ashamed to let others know about my problem. I can't go into the only treatment center nearby; everyone will find out. Besides, my husband and his family are prominent and well-known members of this small community. It would cause them great humiliation."

The fear of public scrutiny and condemnation is a powerful deterrent to seeking addiction treatment. Eve, a single working mother, provides another example of this fear. She told the group, "I can't risk tarnishing my image as a mother or employee by entering a rehab center. God knows I look at the place every time I drive by and wish that I could just walk in and say, 'HELP ME!'"

Any recovering addict can sympathize deeply with her fear. I have felt the same and did not overcome it on my own. Yet I know that sooner or later her drug addiction will tarnish her image much more than entering a drug rehabilitation facility would ever do. Besides, the self-respect she can gain through recovery will be much more real and joyful than the image she tries to project while addicted.

The previous examples of different types of denial were meant to enlighten. Anyone suffering with addiction likely sees him or herself in one or many of the stories shared. What addicts must do is forget "but I can't" thoughts. Telling yourself treatment is "not an option" is absurd. Consider the option you have chosen instead: abusing prescription or over-the-counter medications. Thinking, "I can't risk" treatment is dangerous. Consider the risks you have decided to take by abusing drugs: jail, sickness, disability, loss of family/job, death. How could treatment possibly be riskier than that?

As for the cost of going into treatment or difficulties of finding childcare, these are certainly real concerns. However, there are many options to choose from, some more affordable than others, some providing more flexibility than others. Have you researched all of your options? Very few of those who use excuses like, "I can't take time off from work" or "I don't have anyone to take care of the kids" have actually explored the options that are available (e.g. leaves of absence, use of sick days, the cost of nannies vs. group child-care, company funded childcare). The cost of an absence from work or of twenty-four-hour childcare for a few weeks or months while you are in treatment is high, but probably minimal compared to the cost of your habit over a year's time. Think about what you spent on drugs last month. And what will you do about money and childcare if you end up in jail? Stop saying you can't. Forget "not an option." The fact is you can, as many have done. Including me. Parents, other relatives or friends can sometimes help out with your children, many companies offer leaves of absence, loans and credit card debts can eventually be paid off and you can live on less for a while.

The first time denial begins to drop away is not the time to relax. Denial doesn't instantly disappear. Denial for prescription addicts must be peeled away in layers like leaves of an artichoke. But the process is different for each person. For example, at first, you may admit your problem to yourself, but deny it to others—or the other way around. At some point, perhaps when caught in the act, you may admit your problem to others, casting off the tough outer leaves of denial. But even then, you may secretly think you are different from other prescription addicts and deny the impact of your addiction on your life and the lives of those around you. Every leaf of denial must be peeled away until they are all gone. It is not a quick or simple process. But it can be done.

If you have told yourself that you are finished with denial and are ready to be honest, but you haven't reached the point that you can tell someone else, try your story out on God or some other spiritual entity. As long as this higher power has meaning for you, speak to it. Get your feelings out. Enjoy sharing without interruption or criticism.

If you're not spiritual or are not quite ready for God, write out your thoughts in a journal or try your confession out on the most understanding, imaginary person you can fabricate. Practice your spiel in bed, in the shower or in the car. It doesn't really matter where, just as long as it's peaceful, quiet and safe from the scrutiny of others. Know that this imaginary person, like God, will understand and care. If you can begin peeling back the layers of denial, even just a little, you are ready to get help from an appropriate person. This person—whether it be a psychologist, counselor or support group sponsor—is a real human being who will talk to you in the same understanding way that you imagined, someone who will talk to you in a way that gives you hope and support. An understanding professional therapist, a treatment center staff member, a social worker somewhere in your community is waiting to help you right now. Make the call. And keep reading.

> > > 3

ADMITTING THE PROBLEM:
"That's when I knew I needed help."

Wwhat makes people finally face the disease of prescription addiction? One recovering prescription abuser explains, "When I exhausted myself with pills and over-the-counter drugs and then became severely depressed, I had to make a decision whether to live or lie down and die."

"When you've gone so low in your life that up is the only direction you can go," responds another.

It's often said that you don't reach a turning point in addiction until you have hit rock bottom. Yet "rock bottom" has a different meaning for each person. Sometimes it means the loss of a marriage and family; other times it's loss of professional standing; it can also be lying sick on the floor; and sometimes it's feeling extreme shame. "Rock bottom" usually involves the loss of whatever is most important to you. Sometimes addicts don't actually identify their "rock bottom" on their own. It may happen that a confrontation by a spouse or family member gets the person into treatment. Unfortunately for some, it may take an encounter with the police. Any of these forms of hitting the bottom may propel you towards recovery. Each route has its own elements, its own twists and turns. But you don't have to wait until you hit the bottom. Experiencing vicariously the turning points of others who have gone before you could inspire you to make changes in your life. Give it a chance.

Let's start with those who were forced to face their problem by others. Notice the common thread in each story: "I got caught, they demanded, I was forced, I lost my job, they gave me an ultimatum." If only it didn't come down to being forced to face their addictions, imagine the anguish these individuals and their loved ones could have avoided. No one wants to spend a night in jail or have their spouse threaten divorce, but for some, it takes such drastic measures to make them not only face their addictions, but jump-start their desire to live a sober, drug-free life.

*I didn't start to pay the consequences until my husband noticed I was having memory and weight loss, as well as a personality change. **He insisted** I call my therapist and fill her in on all my self-medicating escapades.*

*My turning point came when **I lost my job** and found that **others knew** I had a problem.*

*I **got caught** eleven days ago by my fellow workers at the hospital. I was so embarrassed, but they did not call the authorities and have kept it pretty quiet. Actually, I felt very much relieved when this intervention took place.*

As the previous anecdotes reveal, the embarrassment of getting caught or the loss of a job can be the jolt one needs. Though pressure from friends or family may not force everyone to a turning point, a serious ultimatum might, as the next story reveals.

*One afternoon, my father called **demanding to know** what was going on with me. Later that same day, my husband told me **he was ready to leave me. They both told me to make a choice**. My father hit home with the children and my husband. I knew I had to do something. I told my doctor, who referred me to a psychiatrist and addictionologist. That day, I called and made an appointment. It was the best thing I ever did.*

Another prescription addict who was turned around by her family's ultimatum shared the following story.

*My husband went behind my back and talked to a family therapist. **They gave me an ultimatum:** either I checked into a treatment center or my husband would leave me and take the kids. I broke down and just wanted to die for putting my babies at harm. Luckily, I had great counselors at the treatment center who helped me get in touch with my feelings and deal with life on life's terms. I also get great support from my involvement with Narcotics Anonymous. It helps knowing there are others out there who have lived and survived this hellish nightmare.*

The turning point for Kim, twenty-five, came when she was caught by someone less sympathetic than kindly employers or family members.

Hitting my "bottom" was the night my home was searched by police who suspected I was dealing prescription drugs. This was not true; I was having a very hard time keeping a supply for myself. **I was forced** *to go to an inpatient treatment center. There I prayed that God would help me and send caring people to my aid. God did send the caring people of Narcotics Anonymous and the wonderful counselors at the treatment center where I got help.*

As Kim's account clearly reveals, those who don't respond to concerned family members or unhappy employers can expect more drastic interventions. Several support group members who went through experiences similar to Kim's shared with me the next shocking stories.

My uncontrollable addiction was so strong that while inside the pharmacy I used to take a look at other people's prescriptions that were laying on the counter. Then I would get in my car and pull up to the drive-thru and tell the pharmacist I was picking up a prescription for whatever name I had seen on the counter and they would give it to me. **I was caught** *by the DEA soon after with heavy fines and a jail sentence.*

Another young woman got the message and got off light. She's now in recovery.

I hit bottom when I lost a boyfriend, my job, my family's trust and was almost arrested three different times for falsifying a prescription. The third time, I was taken by officers to the police station. There they told me the severity of the offense (I had no idea it was Federal) and demanded that I obtain help. Today, I feel lucky to be where I am: clean, sober and not in prison.

Addicts forced into treatment often fail because they didn't make the decision to get help on their own and thus are unable to commit to change. However, this is not always the case, as told in the next story in which forced treatment had an especially happy ending.

Eventually, having worn out my welcome just about everywhere, I started calling in my own prescriptions. **I soon got caught**. *Over the next three years, I spent a total of seven months in jail and went through three* rehab programs. My turning point came after three and a half months in jail when I was sent to a state-run rehabilitation facility. It was truly a special place. There, I met a fellow recovering addict. When we were released, we decided to try living together. It has been two years since I got clean. I have a job I like and a fulfilling relationship with my fellow recovering addict. We now have a six-month-old baby.

Joanna, a young woman with a successful career in the financial industry, also shares the story of her turning point.

I was arrested at a drugstore for trying to pass a forged prescription. I was taken to the city's police station, where I sat for several hours until I was transferred to the county facility. During that time, I was going through withdrawal and, even though I was facing a major felony charge, the only thing I could think of was getting drugs. I was released when a friend put his house up for bail. That day I made a decision that I could not live like that anymore. I was able to check into a detox hospital and went through hell for several days. During that time I was introduced to Narcotics Anonymous. I was shocked to learn that other people actually had stories like mine! The most important thing I learned was that I was not alone! I recently celebrated my fifth anniversary with Narcotics Anonymous. I am very grateful to be alive today.

The following story from a thirty-nine-year-old addict paints a vivid picture of how devastating and life-changing hitting bottom can be.

One day, as I sat waiting for the doctor in an exam room—under the fake name I had been using—the door to the room opened and the police walked in. **I was arrested**, handcuffed and led out of the doctor's office through a busy waiting room with everyone staring at me. They searched my belongings and found evidence of every doctor I had ever seen under the name I made up. Each prescription I received under my fake name from different doctors was a separate felony charge. I was booked on seven class C felony charges. I had never so much as had a speeding ticket before and now I was headed straight to jail. I spent six days in jail before I could see the judge and post bail. In jail, they don't care how sick you are due to withdrawal. I lost twelve pounds in three days from vomiting. I am now on supervised release, which means I have a case manager to whom I must report every week. I have to call the corrections department every day to see if I have come up for a random urine sample. This can happen up to three times a week. I cannot take pain medication anymore regardless of the fact that I have a documented *medical condition that causes me great pain. I just have to live with it. I became addicted and broke the law, so now I must suffer.*

As the previous stories indicate, it would be much better to make the decision to turn around by yourself instead of waiting for the police to come knocking on your door. On the one hand, you could reduce the amount of time you spend sick and miserable. You might also avoid dealing with the justice system, alienating your family and losing the trust of just about everyone you know.

What follows are stories of people who saw the writing on the wall and faced their problems voluntarily, before it cost them their families, jobs or freedom. In a way, it was harder for them, because they had to find the courage within to take that first step. But courage has its rewards as Linda reveals in the next story.

Telling my husband about my addiction after being married only three months terrified me. I feared that he would leave me. When I finally got up the courage to tell him, he was very supportive and understanding. Together we went to see an addictionologist-therapist to help start my treatment. My husband and I went to counseling together and also individual therapy to work out our own issues on recovery.

Another woman, Carol, wasn't able to be as open about her addiction with her spouse or family members. However, the strong, healthy mental state she had before her addiction developed helped her solve her problem rationally and on her own. Carol had a long time addiction to painkillers as a result of breaking her back and other injuries sustained in a horrible car wreck. Actually, after the initial healing, a chiropractor was keeping her tolerably comfortable, but when the insurance would no longer pay for the chiropractic treatment, she went to a physician who gave her painkillers. She found them so pleasurable, she started taking extra doses. After years of escalating tolerance, she was taking ten to fifteen 7.5 mg. tablets of Lortab a day plus 2 mg. of Xanax to calm her. She threw in some other pills whenever the opportunity arose, sometimes not knowing what they were.

For many years, Carol's divorced mother had a constant companion, a kind man whom Carol thought of as her second father. His heavy drinking had not really been a problem in the relationship, but slowly his health and body were being destroyed by his habit. His final illness due to alcoholism was terrible to watch and his death devastated Carol and her mother. As she explains, the loss of this father figure became a turning point for Carol.

I thought, if daily doses of alcohol can do this to a strong, vibrant man, what are all the painkillers doing to my body? Then I began to think about what would happen if I was in another car accident and was injured or if I had to have another operation. The doctors would give me painkillers, but in doses much lower than I needed just to get up in the morning. My tolerance for painkillers was so high, I'd need much more than the doctors would give me. I'd have to confess to my addiction. Or, even worse, maybe I would be unconscious and the doctors would operate on me thinking I was anesthetized when in reality I could feel every painful moment.

These fears of pain and death haunted her, so she began to think of a way out.

Instead of thinking, *I have to have this pill,* she began thinking, *A long time ago I was dealing with my pain without painkillers. My chiropractor was all I needed. If I could get along without pills way back then, I should be able to get along without them now.*

And so Carol began her recovery with these realistic, truthful thoughts instead of the blindness of denial.

Another woman, Susan, was very much in denial, claiming to lead a picture perfect life with a husband, three kids and devotion to her church. She also, however, had a group of friends, wives and mothers like herself, who traded prescription pills. Here's the story of what finally helped her break out of denial and see the truth.

This past week I took pills from a friend not even knowing what they were. I just knew it was some sort of narcotic and I had to take it. This made me realize just how desperate I am. I know that I am no different than the person buying drugs on the street. For years I've fooled myself into thinking it's okay because they are "prescription." Realizing all this made me seek help.

Like Linda, Carol and Susan, many people who take that first step on their own do so because of some major crises or turning points in their lives. The following two brief stories from recovering or soon-to-be recovering addicts relate their jolting moments.

My son asked me if he could have a new bike, but I didn't have the money because I had just spent it on Vicodin. That's when it hit me that I was putting my life and my family on hold for this drug. I knew then that I had to stop.

Little did I know what I was getting myself into! Two years later and many thousands of dollars wasted, I realized that I had to stop. I could not afford the medication without bankrupting my family's savings. So I went to my family doctor and told him about my problem. He was very understanding and referred me to a drug clinic. I am starting detox tonight—finally!

I conned so many pills from a friend with chronic pain that she was cut off by her doctor for using too many pills every month. Now she is up the creek without a paddle and really needs the OxyContin for terrible pain. She has never abused them. Also, I spent all of the "emergency" money in my bank account on OxyContin—three to four pills a day at sixty dollars a pill. It went real fast! I am now about to start a detox program and I am petrified of going through the withdrawal symptoms, but I know this is for the best.

The next story, told by Leslie, describes a more dramatic deliverance from denial and addiction than most of us can expect. Yet, it can happen, as Leslie explains.

Between 1994 and 1999 I lost nine jobs, had four cars repossessed, lost friends, lost boyfriends and overdosed in my bathroom with my little son in the house with me. It is only by the grace of God that I didn't die right there in front of him. Finally, I was ready to end it all after another breakup with the third emotionally abusive boyfriend in a row. I thought I was worthless. I hated myself and believed that I was a complete failure who couldn't change. I prayed and asked God to help me. When I got no answer, I figured He didn't hear me and didn't care. Though I didn't care about dying, I feared what would happen to my little boy, whom I loved greatly, if I took my own life. So I decided to give God one "last chance." Then, if He didn't answer me, I was going to kill myself or die of an overdose.

Less than three months later, I experienced the best day of my life. A miraculous event took place one night that changed the course of my life forever. On that day, I went to a service at my sister's church. I was drawn there like a magnet. I never went to church—much less on a weekday. Anyway, the preacher said a special prayer for me. The moment he finished, I fell to the floor, forced down by some unseen force. I felt hot and my whole body went numb. Everything faded around me. Then came the sound of the sweetest man's voice that I had ever heard. He said, "I had to take it from you—it was going to kill you." I felt certain it was God speaking to me. He delivered me of drugs and alcohol that night and changed my life. It was not a magic wand or anything—though it seemed like it at the time. I have relapsed a few times, but I get stronger every day. I am not perfect—but I am a thousand times better than I was two years ago.

Although Henry did not have the dramatic experience Leslie recounts, in the next story he tells how letting go of denial set him on the path to recovery. He's not completely recovered yet, but he's well on his way.

The turning point for me was last October. I had come home from work and my long-time girlfriend (with whom I have a small son) had found evidence of my addiction while cleaning up the house and confronted me about it. I couldn't lie to her anymore. I told her the whole story of how I had started and stopped on and off several different times. At the time she caught me, I was not even actively taking the pills she found. She was very forgiving and said that she would do everything she could to help me through this. But soon afterwards, I started abusing the drug again and this time I could barely go a day without it. I came to her and told her I was back on it and this time decided to tell my parents. They were disappointed, but they wanted to help me. I was able to go a few days without the drug, but I soon started taking it again. Finally, I went to a drug rehabilitation center for some professional help. I have done pretty good so far, but it is an ongoing battle.

Barry, thirty-two, addicted to painkillers, found a miracle in the fellowships of Narcotics and Alcoholics Anonymous. As most recovering addicts do, Barry has relapsed; however, he's not giving up.

Once I realized that my best thinking got me into a huge mess, I began really listening to what the people at the meetings had to say. They all said the same things! They had done the terrible things I had done to get drugs...manipulating, stealing, lying and the list goes on. They had denied their problem, they had tried to "fix" themselves and they had repeatedly failed. They had lived through the same loneliness and fear as I was still experiencing. These peaceful, happy faces at the Narcotics Anonymous and Alcoholics Anonymous meetings had been where I was—and made it out. I realized I was not alone and I didn't have to do it alone. I have stayed clean for nearly three years. They have been the best three years of my life!

Love of children is an important motivator for those who voluntarily seek recovery. Beth, who only recently admitted to having a problem, cites her child as the biggest factor in her turn-around.

In the past, I have spent as much as $200 or more on pills in a week. My daughter should be the center of our world, but she isn't. She deserves better.

I am at a turning point. I realize that it is the simple things in life that will make me happy: having my child close to me and being clean and sober.

The next inspirational story should be of help to Beth or anyone struggling with addiction. It demonstrates how wonderful it can feel to unburden yourself of addiction by sharing your secret with others and receiving much needed help and support.

I think the turning point came when I ran out of my prescription again (this had happened a lot). This time I still had two weeks to wait for a renewal and I went through a terrible withdrawal period, worse than any other time. I also remembered what the doctor had said about the amount I was already taking. It was on a Saturday when it all finally became clear to me or at least as clear as you can be when you are addicted to narcotics. I started crying and didn't stop for days. I admitted everything to my husband that night and to the rest of my family the next day. First thing on Monday morning I called my doctor's office crying uncontrollably and said I had to come and see him. My husband and I went in that morning and I told my doctor everything as well. He informed me that he suspected this was happening and told me he was proud of me and respected me for telling him and my family. He assured me that he was going to help. He said he felt that he was partially to blame for what had happened and that he just wanted to help me with the headaches and honestly didn't know what else to do after we had tried so many things.

While voluntary treatment seems like a more committed way to seek recovery than being hauled off by the police, choosing to stop taking drugs on your own also means you can choose to return to drugs pretty easily. Ronda made her choice—or has she? At the very least, she has taken the first step of admitting she has a problem and asking for help.

Today I told my husband. He is very supportive. I have twenty pills left which I gave to him so I can get off of them this time without going through withdrawal symptoms. My husband is going to give me one every eight hours. But I have three refills remaining on this prescription and I really do want this to be the end—but I know, if I want to, I can go get them refilled.

If one bad thing occurring doesn't motivate you to stop living in denial, perhaps two bad things happening in one week will hit home, as the next story reveals.

I never admitted to anyone or myself that I was an addict. Then a close friend broke down one day and cried for me to get help. I was shocked she knew what I was doing. Then, in that same week, I called a doctor at home trying to get pills and he confronted me about my addiction. I was so ashamed that I ever let it get so carried away.

Whether the motivating moment to face addiction comes about because of concern for the well-being of a beloved child, fear of physical harm or worry about finances or jail, every addict has his or her own priority. One young woman, Amanda, places physical appearance and beauty high atop her priority list. It was this vanity that both lead to her addiction and ultimately motivated her to stop abusing prescription drugs.

My addiction started after I got breast implants. I took painkillers for a year and a half. A few weeks ago, I woke up and realized I had no more pills left. I looked at the complexion of my face and freaked out. I usually have a perfect complexion, but over the past six months it has gotten terrible. I believe it is because of the medication. I have quit cold turkey. So far, it's been okay; support from my fiancé and my mother has helped a lot. It has also helped to see my complexion clear up and return to normal. Even more important than that, I have discovered peace of mind.

Joelle was able to admit she had a problem and move towards getting help. Her tale seems to sum up all the reasons addicts discover for finally seeing the light.

It is because of my guilt, the fear of what I am doing to my organs, the fear that I will get into trouble for getting these prescriptions refilled so many times and my need to be free of this, that I am going to do whatever it takes to beat this once and for all.

While there may be one point at which an addict gives up denial, usually there are several points. As you may have noticed, in several individuals' stories in this book, including mine, there is a statement along the lines of "that's when I knew I had a problem." Then later in the same story, a statement like, "That's when I *really* knew I had a problem" appears. Even further down there's often the claim, "That's when I knew I needed help." Just as the layers of denial are slowly peeled away, so is the dawn of truth something that usually comes in episodes. While some people experience a "miraculous" moment that immediately pushes them to seek help, most experience several small epiphanies, each leading one step closer to full admission of the problem and reaching out to those who can help.

Shawna (see chapter 1), who had surgery as a very young girl and became addicted to pain medicine, sought unnecessary surgery by faking pain in order to get drugs and relieve stress in her life. Shawna's first moment of casting off denial was by no means her last moment of denial. It took many years and much suffering to admit the whole truth and get help. Still, the first step taken in seeking assistance lays the foundation necessary to build on. Here's more of Shawna's story:

Before each surgery, I would sometimes wish that I would never wake up. I knew the risks involved each time and I was completely ready to take them. What kind of life was this? Faking pain to get drugs. Undergoing invasive surgeries just to get psychological relief. Even through all this, I would tell myself, "It's okay...the doctor's in charge." I still didn't know what an addict was. Meanwhile, I was being touted as a "spiritually strong young lady." I was being admired for enduring so much and with a smile.

Well, the next semester came and I signed up for courses again. This time I could only go a couple of weeks before the need for relief was unbearably strong. Another abdominal attack. My roommates rushed me to the ER. I was admitted and on the operating table in no time at all. Something happened to me that day as I was being prepped for surgery...you could call it an awakening or a voice from God. But I could see exactly what I was doing for the first time. I started feeling cold and clammy and I knew that if I went through with the surgery, I would die that day.

I told the doctor, "I'm sorry, but I can't have this surgery."

He looked perplexed. "What do you mean?"

"I'm sorry, I can't explain. Just please don't put me under."

"Okay," he replied, "but your parents won't be happy. They're going to be charged for it anyway."

My parents were livid and made me come home from college. Their insurance refused to cover any of the bill, which left them owing the hospital $5,000. How could I blame them for being so angry? This caused me to go deeper and deeper into depression.

Shawna at last knew what she was doing. Being sent home to angry parents with forty painkillers in her pocket, however, was not a prescription for recovery as we will see in later chapters.

Reading this book could be your first step away from denial or your seventeenth. However, when you have read these stories with tears of sympathy, fear of the same suffering the tellers of these candid accounts experienced and longing for the happy endings some of them now have, hopefully you will decide it's time for you to let go of the last vestige of your own denial—and take the next step.

Perhaps you fear that your friends and co-workers will treat you differently if you admit you're a prescription addict. I understand the fear. Some people may be surprised to hear you had a problem with prescription addiction, mainly because they have never heard of this type of addiction before and they've never seen you pop a handful of pills. But once you begin to tell your story, if you choose to honestly tell *all* your story, they will respect you even more for coming forward and being candid with them. Others that you are closest to will be glad to see the difference in you and will support you in every way.

And what about your family? Your family may be shocked to learn the truth or relieved to put a name on the problems they have been observing in you for quite a while. Then, in all likelihood, they will be proud of you for coming forth and admitting to them that you need help. They will support you and try to understand your illness. They will want to help you work through this. True, it will be difficult. Be patient and gentle with them in turn, for some may not be ready to hear everything that needs to be brought to the table. Remember, this isn't easy for them either. Some things take time to mend. You and they will have the time to give each other while you're getting clean and focusing on recovery. Together you all can heal and learn together.

As you want them to forgive you, forgive yourself. Most of us don't always see problems coming until something goes completely wrong. Sometimes, we don't see an oncoming car until it's already too late to avoid a collision. We don't foresee other misfortunes that we wish we could have prevented but had no way of stopping. Why should an unexpected disease be any different? Prescription addiction is a disease, not a character flaw. Some people are more sensitive than others to the effects of addictive medications, including over-the-counter medicines, and may feel euphoric states more intensely. There is also a genetic factor in drug dependence. For a person who is physically addicted, the body's chemical processes are altered so that the drug becomes essential for some of the normal metabolic functions. Prescription addiction is the resulting uncontrollable craving for our drug of choice. This is the tragic truth. Quit beating yourself up about it and start working to change it by reading on and finding out who and where to ask for help.

GETTING HELP:
"Where can I find someone who understands?"

Now that you have said it out loud—"I am addicted and I can't solve my problem by myself"—it's time to seek assistance from people who have the expertise to get you the treatment you need.

The Four Essentials

The four essentials to successfully kicking your prescription drug habit are:
1.) Finding a **treatment center** or other healing environment where you can detoxify;
2.) Obtaining a **therapist**;
3.) Joining a **support group**;
4.) Getting a **sponsor**.

Maybe a few people have succeeded without all four, but they are special cases. You have made a brave decision to beat your addiction. Now give yourself a chance for success: Find all four elements as soon as possible and commit yourself to each of them.

Financing Recovery

I wish money was not an issue when planning addiction recovery, but for many, the first question they worriedly ask themselves is, *Where's the money going to come from?* Your family may be wondering the same thing. Money is an important consideration for almost everyone, so it's necessary to address that matter here.

Hospitalization in some treatment centers can cost $1200 a day or more. Treatment by a psychiatrist as an outpatient usually costs between $100 and $170 per fifty-minute session. Clinical psychologists cost somewhat less, as do other kinds of counseling specialists. Health insurance may cover a large part of treatment in all of these categories. In that case, the more expensive professional treatment covered by insurance may actually cost the individual less money than a cheaper treatment option not covered by health insurance.

Do you have health insurance? If you do, your insurance company can offer a list of treatment facilities that will be covered under your specific plan. They will tell you exactly how many days of treatment they will pay for, based on inpatient or outpatient rehabilitation. Your insurance will also inform you of your choices of therapists to help you with physical and psychological problems.

If you do not have insurance coverage that covers mental healthcare and substance abuse treatment, find out if your community, county or city has a rehabilitation program that is billed on a sliding scale. Look up the name of your county or city in the blue government pages (found between the white and yellow pages) in your telephone book. It's sometimes hard to know what heading is the right one for finding help with addiction recovery because every state, city and municipality seems to use different names for their various services. Look through the listings until you find the Health Department. Under that or separately, look for listings like Alcohol and Drug Treatment, Drug Rehabilitation, Family and Children's Services, individual Health Centers, Mental Health, Social Services, Substance Abuse or Suicide hot line. Look at every heading and call the one most closely related to drug addiction or mental health. Call and ask if they can assist you with substance abuse programs or refer you to a public program that will. Often free healthcare is provided for those whose income and assets are below a certain standard; others charge on a sliding scale according to income. Call and ask what options are available for your recovery needs and income level.

Another option is to call a private treatment center of your choice and ask if someone on the staff can talk to you about financial assistance programs that apply. Or you can contact a large hospital in your area. Ask to talk to the social worker. Most public hospitals have social workers on staff who will talk to you, whether or not you are currently admitted to that hospital. Sometimes you can walk in and find a social worker in her/his office, however, it's better to make an appointment than to show up unannounced and discover the social worker is unavailable to meet with you.

Nonprofit organizations often provide mental health and other services that are billed on a sliding scale. Call the United Way office in your community and ask about these. There may be others that are not affiliated with United Way; you should be able to learn about these, too, if you are persistent in your search.

It may well be that you do not qualify for financial assistance because your income is too high, but you think you cannot afford to pay for extensive medical care for your problem. Considering the alternatives to getting effective treatment, it is obvious that you can't afford NOT to have the necessary medical care for your problem. If it takes you and your family the rest of your lives to pay off the resulting bills, it will be worth it, because it will give you back the rest of your life. Your life is worth it. Your family is worth it. Debt is better than addiction. I know.

1. Find a Treatment Center

If you have been caught, that is, you were found disabled or unconscious and an ambulance was called or you were apprehended doing something illegal, you may have been whisked off to a treatment center without having any choice in the matter. If you came to the conclusion that you needed help by yourself or were persuaded to seek help in a rational moment, then you will have a part in choosing the type of facility in which you will detoxify or "detox." You can obtain a recommendation of a particular drug treatment center by calling your local hospital, asking your primary physician or one of his staff members, by personal recommendation or, if you have the opportunity, by going to several facilities to look them over and ask questions. If you truly have no one you can ask, look in the yellow pages of your telephone directory under Drug Treatment for a list of treatment centers. Alternatively, you may choose to detox at home. If you do so, I urge you to seek out a therapist first, one who will guide you in making the decision about how and where to detox. Unfortunately, most addicts who seek help do so in a crisis situation in which they must make quick decisions with little information. If you are in such a situation, try to contact an informed person—like a doctor or therapist—for assistance first.

In my own case, I had been lost on a highway and finally got home with my face numb from overdose. I felt as if I was having a stroke. Frightened,

I called the toll-free telephone number printed on the back of my insurance company card labeled "Mental Health/Substance Abuse referral information." I told the person who answered that I was addicted and in bad shape. I asked for the names of professionals in my area whose services would be covered by this insurance. The insurance representative gave me three names and numbers. I telephoned all three. I made an appointment with the only one who could see me that very day. He happened to specialize in child psychiatry, but he did what was best for me. When I showed up in his office, he took my car keys away from me and gave me a choice of being taken to a treatment center by ambulance, the police, my husband or a friend. I chose a friend, because I was too ashamed to face my husband. The psychiatrist himself telephoned my friend and saw to it that I was on my way to a treatment center where he was affiliated. Because he specialized in children, the psychiatrist did not end up being my long-term therapist, but he was a godsend at that turning point in my life.

For those of you who think you want to see a therapist, but do not want to go to a treatment center, you should be aware that if you are in danger of harming yourself and others when you arrive at the therapist's office, the therapist has the legal right to call authorities and force you to go to a treatment center for seventy-two hours in most states regardless of your wishes, and rightly so. If you are driving under the influence of drugs, you are in danger of harming yourself or others. If you go to a therapist in a relatively sober condition, however, you and the therapist together can decide in a more leisurely fashion what kind of treatment options are best for you.

You have the choice of detoxing in a treatment center or at home under the supervision of a psychiatrist. This decision is best made with your physician or therapist, taking into account not only your addictive behavior but your home situation and resources. Those who do not go to a treatment facility must undergo the process of withdrawal with strict supervision by a therapist or physician. The therapist or physician gradually tapers down the dosage of pills to minimize the discomforts of physical withdrawal while requiring frequent follow-up visits. Hospitalization is a surer, more relapse-proof way of detoxing accompanied by more intense medical attention and, usually, by earlier introduction to support groups. It spares your family the stressful experience of your withdrawal. On the next page are charts showing the advantages of receiving care at a treatment facility and the disadvantages of going through withdrawal on your own.

Advantages of Going Through Withdrawal at a Treatment Facility

Medication management
Support groups
Safe environment
Detoxification supervised
Suicide watch
Non-judgmental environment
Vital signs monitored daily
Depression supervised
Not feeling isolated or alone
Changed behaviors learned

Disadvantages of Going Through Withdrawal at Home

No supervision of withdrawal symptoms
Health risks
Depression
Isolation
No guidance or support link
Anxiety
Dangerous environment (triggers)
Confusion and fear
Lack of self-esteem

Those of you who feel you might be the kind of individual who can suc-cessfully kick your drug habit at home or by yourself, remember that while a few addicts have done it, it's hard work and recovery is less certain. Carol, whose comments were shared in chapter 3, is one fortunate individual who succeeded in this difficult endeavor.

Carol's Story

During my forty-one years of life I have learned that a human being has many faults and many strengths. There have been many trials and tribulations in my life that have tested my inner strength. This will be the first time I tell my story to anyone. I never told my husband or my family about my pill addiction in fear of judgement and criticism.

I was driving home one bitter, cold December morning with a girl-friend in my small compact car going fifty miles per hour when my left front tire blew out and then approximately twenty seconds later the right front tire blew out. I lost all control of my car. The car began turning in circles on the highway and then rolled over and over, tumbling out of con-trol. During the first roll, my girlfriend, who was sleeping, was thrown out of the passenger door. The door had been locked at the time, but the force of the tumble and of her body broke the door lock and window. She lay prone at the top of the hill and in disbelief watched my car continue to tumble with me still inside. Susan was horrified watching me, her friend, trapped in a vehicle that was being torn apart. It felt like an eternity to me praying for the vehicle to come to a stop. Then, in an instant, I was thrown out the windshield and trapped under the car.

Susan managed to pull herself to the highway with a broken neck and shoulder to flag an eighteen wheeler truck traveling through town. He radioed for an ambulance and police while trying to help Susan. He then made his way down the hill to try to help and comfort me. He asked if he could call someone for me, like my mother. (I was only nineteen and unmarried at the time.) Emergency crews were unable to free me from the wreckage for about ninety minutes. Finally freed, paramedics placed me on a gurney and backboard. Susan and I were able to ride together in the ambulance. It was comforting and reassuring that we were both alive.

Minutes after arrival at the hospital, I was confronted by a very insensitive doctor who told me I would never walk again. My mother arrived at the hospital before we arrived, thanks to the truck driver who called her while we were en route to the hospital. She cried, afraid of my prognosis but grateful I was alive. I have my mother's survival spirit and will to overcome just about anything. I kept this spirit and strength throughout my recovery from a back that was broken in four places and a neck that was broken in two places. My pain was unimaginable and only after many, many hours of X rays and examinations, the doctors finally gave me several types of pain medications. I stayed in the hospital under heavy doses of Morphine and Valium for nine days. I then asked to be tapered off these medications so that I could focus, feel and pull my thoughts together to see what I really could do and not do physically, on my own. I underwent painful physical therapy several times a day, wondering what my real chances would be to walk again or even tie my shoes.

It felt as if every time a doctor came into my room it was with a voice of doom filled with bad news. I chose to tune them out with their negative attitudes and opinions. I told them that I was entirely too young to be paralyzed and, no matter what they said, I would walk again. Susan was discharged from the hospital to continue her recuperation at home with physical therapy. After two weeks in the hospital, I was discharged with the personal determination that I would walk again. During months of physical therapy and living in pain twenty-four hours a day, I made progress. After nearly two years, I was able to walk normally and return to work. I reduced my medications to only a few painkillers a day, but I still felt depressed and anxious.

Two years later, I was told I needed a hysterectomy because of complications from the accident. I was prescribed more painkillers, Lortab, Percodan for back pain and Xanax for anxiety. I became very depressed knowing I could never give birth. I had no one to talk to about my feelings of emptiness and sadness. I was married now, but I could not even talk to my husband about this. My entire life was about helping others in their struggles of pain and emptiness. I learned as a child from an abusive father to keep all emotions bottled inside, not ever asking for help. I was told to fix my own problems and not bother anyone else with them. My best defense was acting the part of a "perfect" child.

Several years went by. I was now abusing the healthcare system, increasing my dosages as I pleased and changing doctors to keep refills promptly supplied. I even convinced myself that if I decreased my pill intake for a few days periodically, this would mean I wasn't an addict. Then I increased again soon after with a larger dose. I convinced myself I was always in control, not realizing my pills were controlling me.

The reality of addiction struck me one day when another friend and I were watching a movie at the theatre; we swapped pills like people sharing popcorn or candy. We both laughed as we swallowed pills not even knowing what the pill was and we didn't care about the consequences we could have faced. It didn't even matter what movie was being shown, only getting high mattered. Suddenly it turned sour. I drove home in tears thinking it really wasn't funny or fun anymore. I had become no better than any other addict needing a fix to feel better about myself. If I wanted to be a better person, I had to do the work...alone. I wasn't ready to share my misery with anyone!

I called my medical insurance first, but they wouldn't cover inpatient treatment or counseling. My second call was to my neurologist, who had written my recent prescriptions for pain medications, to inform him that I wanted to get off all medications, that I had become dependent on them and that I needed his help to gradually decrease the dosages. I was honest with him about all the substances I was abusing, including an over-the-counter sleep aid. He reassured me he heard stories of prescription addiction every day and that the number of patients complaining of their misuse increases every year. Without hesitation, he worked out a treatment plan with me. He prepared me for possible side effects of decreasing my doses after my body had become accustomed to much higher amounts. He tried to convince me to talk to my husband or mother about my problem, but I couldn't. I replied I was too ashamed, embarrassed and angry to reveal my weakness. Emotionally, I always felt pills were my survival link to living a normal life. Pills kept me feeling balanced and normal (I thought); without them, I would crumble and lose control of everything I worked so hard to get back since my accident. Once again, I turned to my inner strength, praying for guidance to pull me through this, as I had to do this for myself and for no one else.

Even with excellent guidance from my doctor in tapering my doses, I began to feel the effects of withdrawal within two days. I felt edgy and irritable and had difficulty with concentration. After one week, I was getting up in the middle of the night with sweats and throwing up, classic withdrawal symptoms. My husband and I were arguing over the littlest things. He was unhappy that I didn't want to join in the activities I used to enjoy when I was on pills. He would go out on the boat for a ten-hour day. I just knew I couldn't sit on a boat with him and a dog for ten hours without going nuts. My husband noticed, of course, and while he was still unaware of my condition, he was showing concern about what might be wrong. I isolated myself from family and friends, fearing they might guess what was wrong. By the second week, my withdrawal symptoms were lessening, but I was severely depressed, still not able to confide in anyone or even wanting to.

After three weeks, I returned to work, which helped me focus on something else and forget my own troubles. I began a regimen of exercises at home and joined a gym to alleviate stress. I was told exercise can help sweat out the toxins in my system faster. Even though my withdrawal symptoms lasted on and off for about six months, after four weeks I could function daily without disruptions in my day.

My withdrawal symptoms finally ceased, but I knew I needed to talk to someone about the emotional distress I had buried for years. More importantly, I needed support. I needed someone to whom I could unburden myself of my fears, confusion and shame. I couldn't carry this on my shoulders alone any longer. I went to see my best friend, the one I shared pills with in the theater. She had recently overdosed and nearly died from the same disease I now live with. She was taken into a treatment center and recovered. As I was also recovering, I watched her transform from someone who didn't give a damn whether she lived or died to someone "making a difference," supporting those who feel they also are suffering alone. Her name is Cindy Mogil.

My husband still knows nothing about this. I do not regret not telling him. I honestly think he could not have dealt with it and that would have meant an added strain, perhaps even divorce. As it is, he notices I am a happier person with a good attitude. He just knows he likes the new me better than the old me. That's the way I want to keep it.

Carol's story is a remarkable one. I should add that most of us, including myself, could never have done "the program" at home or without telling a spouse and those closest to us. Also, I must note that, as hard as it is to tell your spouse or other loved ones, getting your addiction out in the open creates a hugely refreshing freedom. You don't walk on eggshells anymore. Your spouse knows the worst, so there is no more fear of the truth from then on. This atmosphere of honesty allows us to build stronger relationships based on trust. I respect Carol's decision; her marriage indeed might not have survived the trauma of her ordeal had her addiction been out in the open. Still, I don't envy her forever carrying this secret at home.

Susan also tells of her abuse of prescription drugs and her desire to recover. She struggled with her addiction to prescription medication for more than twenty-three years.

Susan's Story
I went on vacation in July and as I stood in my hotel room, counting my pills, I looked up and saw myself in the mirror. I knew I had long since

passed the recreational drug use stage. When I returned home and my hus-
band went to work the next day, I began to call treatment centers. They
told me that with the amount of pills I had been taking, it was dangerous
for me to quit cold turkey.

Since I was afraid I'd lose my job if I took any more time off, I went to
my doctor and asked if I could speak to him off the record. He said, "Yes,"
and I told him the WHOLE truth about my abusing prescription drugs and
that I was desperate to quit. He told me I would need to cut back a pill per
day. He also told me I would feel awful. I was up to ten Vicodin a day and
twenty Soma and I really didn't want to spend thirty days detoxing.
Without my doctor's consent, I stopped in five days. It was really rough for
the first couple of weeks. I felt as though I was a child again; I was afraid
of everything. I started going to Narcotics Anonymous and found a meet-
ing group in which most of the members were also addicted to prescription
pills. I got a sponsor and whenever I feel like I am losing my sanity, I reach
out for help. I was also fortunate that in the NA group meeting, a list of
detox side effects was passed out, so I knew what I was going through was
normal.

Whatever road you choose, I am living proof that it can be done. No
matter how rotten you feel as you detox, you never have to feel that way
again if you don't pick up another drug. Life really does get better!

In a way, I am reluctant to tell you about these people who seem to have
kicked their addictions to prescription drugs at home with only moderate
support from doctors and support groups because many, even most, people
cannot succeed this way. I don't want to give unrealistic hope to addicts that
they can recover from drugs without the consequences of anyone knowing.
To some extent, opening up to people and letting them know what you are
going through and experiencing a healing process with them is the essence
of recovery. In the chapter on denial I have even described the excuse,
"treatment in a treatment center is not an option," as a form of denial. It is
rare that an excuse for not entering a treatment center is reasonable or rational. However, the next story gives one reason that is chilling.

I just decided to get off pills two days ago. Although I was only on three
pills a day, withdrawal still hurts badly. I went to a clinic to get help and
they turned me away. They said I had to be on a minimum of at least
twenty pills a day for the past six months. I couldn't believe it. My body
feels like I had been taking thirty pills a day for three years. Even at three

*pills a day, I feel withdrawal symptoms that are just killing me. I am hop-
ing that this is the worst of it.*

In support group meetings and on-line chatroom discussions, caring people urge others to seek outside help with statements like, "You can't quit at
home. I know. I've tried it numerous times." And even of those who have quit
on their own at home, many aren't successful at maintaining long-term sobriety without the education and total care a treatment center provides. After all,
quitting is not the same as *recovery*. As one recovering addict put it, "Quitting
is not the real problem. It's just a bad week and lots of Tylenol. I've done it many
times. The real problem is finding a way to get off and stay off drugs."

If you have made the big step to get help at a treatment center, either by
yourself or with a therapist's recommendation, you will be "assessed" there
by a staff psychiatrist or other staff counselor to plan the best treatment plan
for you. If you have a therapist, his or her recommendations will be included
in your treatment plan as well since he or she knows your history and you
have already established a relationship with someone you trust.

A complete assessment involves being asked a number of questions. It is
to your advantage to answer these honestly and completely. You will be asked:

> To provide medical history.
> To provide your history of prescription abuse, including over-the-
counter medicines and any other mood-altering substances.
> To provide your patterns of abuse (use everyday, night, morning,
afternoons?).
> How much and how many pills you take everyday.
> What your drug of choice is.
> What other types of drugs and intoxicants (e.g. mixing with other
medications or alcohol) you use.
> How you are functioning psychologically, educationally, occupation-
ally, spiritually, socially, interpersonally and recreationally.
> How you are obtaining your pills (e.g. from your family physician or
dentist, through forgeries, by calling in your own refills or someone
else's, by multiple unnecessary surgeries, from the Internet or stealing from emergency rooms, friends or family members.)
> How much money you spend on prescriptions and over-the-counter
medicines per month.
> If you have any blackouts, memory loss or withdrawal symptoms.

As the assessment progresses, the "interviewer" will be observing you for any mood, anxiety, personality or other disorders you may be unconsciously exhibiting. He will also be observing your physical appearance, behaviors and how you interact with others who may be with you during your assessment meeting.

The interviewer will ask about family members who also may have a substance abuse dependency or psychiatric illnesses, since many mental disorders tend to run in families like any other disease.

The treatment facility, in my experience, is the best place, maybe the only place, to detoxify your body and go through withdrawal from drugs. This process is discussed again in great detail in chapter 6.

2. Obtain a Therapist (psychiatrist, addictionologist, psychologist, counseling social worker)

You may have chosen a therapist before coming to the treatment center. Do you still trust and have confidence in this therapist? Do you feel he or she understands addiction and has the necessary knowledge and experience? If so, you are set. If not, you can change.

Or perhaps the treatment center has assigned a therapist to you. Certainly you can accept or veto this choice or you can try the recommended therapist for a while. If it doesn't work out, you can always change, believe me.

In my case, the treatment center assigned me a psychiatrist. He may have provided excellent care for others, but he didn't help me at all. When he asked me if I was sleeping well and I said "not at all," he prescribed Ativan. Ativan is very addictive, which I well knew, but I was a sick person so I said, "Fine." He said he was going to give me ten pills to help me sleep for ten nights, then he told me to come back in two weeks. When he actually wrote the prescription, however, out of habit he wrote it for thirty days. My relapse was sealed right there. This doctor, to give him the kindest judgment, did not understand addiction and the journey one needs to take to reach recovery.

When I returned to the treatment center in relapse and had detoxed again, I was in an "after-care" group. This is a group which meets at the hospital under the guidance of a trained counselor. There I got a recommendation for a psychiatrist who truly understands addiction. It was Dr. Angela Cornell, who proved to be excellent for my needs and whom I still see today on occasion. She is also the person who wrote the preface to this book.

You need a therapist with training and experience with addiction, but more important than credentials, in my opinion, is a recommendation by someone in recovery who has successfully used the therapist. One good place to find such a recommendation is a support group.

3. Join a Support Group

If you have been in a treatment facility, you will probably have been introduced to support groups almost immediately, although you may not have participated. You may be required to go and, even if you go reluctantly, you will soon see how valuable they are. You will discover what being truly honest really means. You will discover others have the very same feelings you have. Later, you may also be in an "after-care" group, which is part of your treatment even though it will be on an outpatient basis. After-care groups are guided by a counselor.

When you are released from the treatment center, you will be given the names, places and times for support groups in your area. These may include chapters of Narcotics Anonymous (NA), Alcoholics Anonymous (AA), or Prescription Anonymous. The last organization was not in existence when I was released and, while I found AA and NA helpful and even critical, something was missing—people who had similar experiences to mine. There was no group that could share with me the special circumstances of prescription addiction. That is absolutely why I founded Prescription Anonymous in Atlanta and have worked hard to sponsor groups in other communities around the country. In any case, there are many reasons to utilize all of the relevant groups within your reach. First, you will need frequent meetings in the early weeks and months after your treatment. Second, since every group has a different perspective, different people and a different "feel," it takes time to find a group you are comfortable with. After you've visited several different group meetings, you can decide with your therapist which groups you do not need or like and choose the one that best fits your needs as you embark upon the road to recovery.

For me, attending meetings will be a lifetime activity that provides the ongoing support I need. However, if I find that the meetings of one group become too repetitive or unhelpful, I simply go to other meetings. These groups are flexible and forgiving. You will not be criticized if you suddenly decide a particular meeting isn't working for you. You will also be welcomed without judgment when you attend a meeting for the first time, yet you won't be forced to participate any more than you'd like to. It is for these reasons that I strongly urge recovering addicts to not only attend support group meetings in the beginning, but to continue attending for the rest of their lives. As a lifelong activity, it will foster lifelong recovery.

If, for any reason, contact information for support groups is not given to you by your treatment center or therapist, you can call any of the national organizations listed in appendix II and ask for contact information for chapters in your area. You can also look up these groups by name in the white pages of the telephone book or look for Support Groups in the yellow pages where you may find other appropriate local groups. I hope to soon have Prescription Anonymous listed in phone books nationwide. In the meantime, you can visit the group's Web site at www.prescriptionanonymous.org.

In addition to being members of support groups, many people find the virtual support available on the Internet to be of real value. Such Web sites can be found by visiting Prescription Anonymous' Web page. These Web sites attract stories and comments from people with addiction problems as well as chat rooms where people can anonymously discuss their addictions. Though these sites should not be used as a substitute for proper treatment, the sharing and support may certainly provide some comfort.

4. Get a Sponsor

Sponsorship is a mutual and confidential relationship between two people who are in recovery for similar addictions. The sponsor is a person who has been in recovery for at least a year or two and has the proven skills to maintain sobriety through experience. The sponsor is a special person with whom a new member can discuss personal problems, confusion, anxious moments and uncertainty. The sponsor willingly shares experiences, strength and hope while giving a sense of security. This person contributes the wisdom of his or her experiences in recovery while standing fast and providing stability and seasoned advice as you go through your recovery. The sponsor must also be the same gender as you, because a newly sober addict is emotionally vulnerable to filling the void and pain created in his/her life with a new romantic or sexual interest.

Sponsors are usually found through support groups. If the issue of sponsorship is not mentioned within the group, a new member should feel free to announce that he is looking for a sponsor and ask for recommendations. Sometimes a person willing to be a sponsor may be a regular member of the group. Often the person is not an active member, but is a sponsor to someone else in the group and may also sponsor you if she is willing to take on more than one person at a time. My long-term sponsor had five people under her wing. I am now a sponsor myself. However, two people are all I feel I can help at any given time considering my other commitments. If you cannot find a sponsor through your group, ask your therapist and the staff at a treatment center for recommendations. People willing to be sponsors usually make themselves known to professionals and support groups.

Once you have found potential sponsors, you should interview several to find a person that "clicks" with you. You must be comfortable and able to be honest with this person or you won't call him or her when you should or allow the person to be the best help he or she can be. If the first sponsor you meet doesn't feel right to you, seek another one. Soon after I chose my first sponsor, I decided I needed someone else and changed to a woman on whom I've relied for several years. Don't worry about offending your sponsor if you decide to find someone new. Your sponsor should want what's best for you and be able to part on amicable terms. In fact, often if a connection is not there, your sponsor will sense it as well and won't be surprised when you announce your intention to find a new sponsor. Don't hesitate to do what's in your best interests. The recovery process is too fragile and important for you to depend on the help of an individual with whom you don't share a bond.

The sponsor sets rules that will be most helpful for you and will make the relationship possible for her. It starts somewhat like a business arrangement. The relationship, however, is highly personal. For example, I require those whom I sponsor to call me every day for the first two weeks, because their judgment about when to call is not highly developed. After that I may change the rule. I may say, "I will not manage the program for you. You have to want sobriety enough to seek help every time you need it, not to wait for me to call you or call because I tell you to call."

You may keep the sponsor indefinitely. I am still with mine. I don't call her as often as I used to when I was feeling shaky, of course, but I still touch base with her every couple of weeks. Everyone is different. Some people change sponsors when they need a new perspective; some change every year. Sometimes a new sponsor is in order if you are on a plateau and you think that with a new sponsor, you could refocus on higher goals and move onward. You shouldn't ever be without a sponsor, even if you are not in contact often. You should always have someone you can call on if you need help or reassurance. People tend to relapse if they don't maintain the supportive, nurturing relationship one finds with a sponsor.

Go To Your Primary Care Physician

Now that you have the four essentials in place to help you with recovery, you may wonder about your other "ordinary" healthcare needs. What if you get a sinus infection, pain in your abdomen, a strange rash or any of the many ailments that used to send you to your family doctor? Your psychiatrist isn't going to treat them, is she? Of course not. You'll continue to go to a primary care physician, also called a family practice physician, an internist or general practitioner. It is important that your primary care physician, who perhaps was your doctor before you became addicted to medication, is made aware of your condition.

First, tell your current or original doctor or any new physician, dentist, surgeon, anesthesiologist or other healthcare provider with whom you consult that you suffer from prescription addiction or that you have an addictive personality. This is very important. You must tell **every** healthcare provider you ever see about your addiction.

As for your original or current primary care physician and other doctors and dentists you have seen in the past, ask yourself, was this the doctor under whose care you became addicted? Did he overprescribe medications? Was she a part of your addiction problem or did you do this on your own? Did he ignore the addiction or foster it? Or did you deceive him, hiding your abuse of prescriptions too well? And if she did not foster your addiction, is she knowledgeable about addiction and the latest information about the addictiveness of drugs?

The physician-patient relationship is seriously distorted when either party fails to abide by his or her responsibilities. The American Medical Association (AMA) has developed a categorization for physicians who misprescribe drugs known as "The Four-D Classifications": Duped, Dated, Disabled and Dishonest.

The Duped Physician: A duped physician is one who inadvertently supplies drugs to a prescription addict because the medication abuser posing as a patient has deceived the physician. In this case, it is primarily the patient who has failed to meet his or her responsibility.

Prescription abusers who do not want their drug dependence treated, but rather want access to the medications for which a physician is the gate keeper may create the illusion that they are seeking medical attention for a disease or illness for which the desired drug would be appropriate. Manipulations or scams for medications can be quite sophisticated, innovative and impossible to unravel in the time available for the physician-patient interaction. When patients have used deception to obtain medications or use them in ways other than those prescribed by their physicians, they have violated their responsibility in the physician-patient relationship.

The Dated Physician: Some physicians misprescribe medications because the information on which they base their therapeutic choices is obsolete, incomplete or just plain wrong. Prescribing practices change over time, as new medications become available or as new clinical information and scientific study result in new guidelines. By not keeping abreast of current prescribing practices and of abuse patterns of the prescription addict, out-of-date physicians cannot meet their responsibilities to practice medicine at the same standard as other practitioners in the community. The Dated physician is simply ignorant and has failed to uphold his responsibilities to his patients.

The Disabled Physician: The *American Journal of Psychiatry* showed that rates of chemical dependence in physicians are roughly equivalent to those of the rest of the population; estimates range from 3 percent to 5 percent.[1] Physicians whose judgements are impaired by mental illness, alcoholism or by their own use of psychoactive drugs may prescribe medications irresponsibly to their patients. Moreover, such physicians may withhold from patients medications that are necessary, because these physicians fear that their overall prescribing patterns may draw attention to their own misuse. Disabled physicians breach their responsibilities to their patients, because they do not bring to the physician-patient relationship their best judgment, attention and skill.

The Dishonest Physician: Dishonest physicians are those (less than 1 percent) who use their medical licenses to deal drugs. When a prescription addict consults with a dishonest physician, the physician does not have the patient's well-being in mind as the primary concern. Such physicians are not treating illnesses; they are perpetuating addictions under the guise of legitimate medical practices to avoid prosecution. Dishonest physicians fail to meet their responsibilities to their patients in every possible way.

Physicians who fail in their responsibilities to patients should be censured. The American Medical Association (AMA) in recent years has helped state medical licensing boards and enforcement agencies develop ways of intervening with misprescribing physicians sooner than they used to and with a broader range of options. However, the AMA emphasizes, the current tendencies to assign fault to physicians when patients have violated their responsibilities is unreasonable and unfair to physicians. When patients deceive their physicians or use their medications other than as prescribed, society should hold the patients, not the physicians, accountable for the inevitable adverse consequences.

While writing this book, I received word that my uncle had died. When I heard the whole story, I became angry and more eager than ever to make this book available to the public as soon as possible.

My uncle Tom had been diagnosed as suffering from extreme emotional instability, known as bipolar disorder, for more than forty-five years. His family physician of forty years had prescribed an expensive and potentially dangerous drug called lithium to stabilize his drastic mood swings. Uncle Tom had been in and out of treatment facilities for mental illness most of his adult life with his dear wife of thirty-eight years by his side. Because money was scarce and insurance coverage paid very little, they weren't able to buy all the medicines Tom needed, especially the lithium, which was supposed to be taken on a regular basis. Knowing this, Tom's doctor often came by their house in a little Vermont town to drop off samples of lithium and other medicines, so they rarely needed to purchase prescriptions at the drug store.

Two weeks prior to Tom's death, his doctor died. Tom had to find a new doctor to continue his healthcare. One week after the death of his doctor, Tom found a new family physician. After giving Tom a thorough physical examination, the new physician asked Tom and his wife about his past medical history and inquired about the last time Tom had any blood work done or an overall physical. Tom replied that he had never had blood work or gotten a physical from either his previous doctor in the forty years that he had been treated by him or from any doctor in the many hospitals where he was treated. Tom's new physician was shocked by what he was told and ordered a complete blood workup on Tom. The results were very abnormal, indicating life-threatening health problems. The doctor told Tom that his kidneys were so badly damaged by the ongoing use of lithium and other medications that he couldn't even put Tom on kidney dialysis. The damage was irreversible. Tom passed away at the age of sixty-four, two weeks after his original doctor died. Uncle Tom died from heart and kidney failure, not ever understanding "why."

The causes of the doctor's death make me wonder if the doctor himself was addicted to something. Whether he was *Disabled* or not, he was most certainly *Dated*, practicing outside his area of expertise or grossly negligent. Lithium is known to be a valuable but problematic psychiatric drug. The use of lithium by every standard requires frequent monitoring of kidney function through blood tests. Any sign of a problem indicates the need for an immediate change of treatment. This physician should have been reported to his state board for inappropriate distribution of prescription drugs. Even if no action was taken against him, the inquiry might have made him straighten up and pay attention.

So the question remains: What about your primary care doctor?

If you've been seeing any healthcare professional for a long period of time, you may feel a sense of loyalty to that provider such that the thought of switching to a new doctor seems like an act of betrayal. Even so, you must pay attention to any subtle or gross signs of negligence that may indicate it's time to fire your doctor.[2] This is your right as a patient; your life may depend on it. Ask yourself: *Is my doctor hazardous to my health?*

The following list details six good reasons to fire your healthcare provider. You may come up with additional valid reasons of your own.

Bad Healthcare Providers

> *She always acts rushed.*
If a doctor spends less than three to five minutes with you, it may be because the bottom line or corporate regulation is on her mind, according to Jamie Court, co-author of *Making a Killing: HMO's and the Threat to Your Health*. "Doctors have a fixed budget for each patient...The result of this reimbursement system—known as capitation—is that the less they do for you, the more money they make." Doctors have an incentive to take on more patients while spending less time with each of them. "Unfortunately, when you speed up the conveyor belt," says Court, "there are bound to be more errors."[3]

> *He displays inappropriate behavior.*
Inappropriate touching can range from lingering too long over the breasts or genitals during an examination to an unnecessary rectal exam. The question here is how comfortable you feel with what your doctor is doing. Is there a second person in the room with you, such as a nurse or assistant, while the examination is being conducted? You can insist on it. Unacceptable behavior can also include verbal comments such as: "You're my last patient of the day so I'm free after this," or "You're cute." Innuendo or suggestive jokes should not be made at any time during the examination. Sometimes behavior that seems inappropriate to a younger adult will not bother an older adult, because he or she and the doctor are from a generation where such behavior may have been commonplace. However, don't chalk up a doctor's inappropriate behavior or comments to generational differences. If your doctor makes you feel uncomfortable or uneasy, even if you can't put your finger on why—it may be time to find someone new.

> *She talks down to me.*
Even though you may not have a medical degree, you shouldn't be made to feel as if you're too inadequate to understand your diagnosis. The doctor shouldn't withhold information because "You won't be able to understand

it." Usually, it is a good idea to ask for clarification in simple language when you don't understand and to jot down technical names and medical terms used in diagnoses. This way, should you decide to go to the library to research your illness or should you change doctors, you'll be able to report your diagnosis to your new physician.

> He is not open to alternative health solutions.
Some doctors have extreme difficulty believing in alternative health solutions such as chiropractic or herbal medicine or newer medical measures he's not familiar with. Debates with your physician on these topics can lead to bad feelings and serious complications in your relationship. If you can't accept or believe in your physician's approach to your healthcare needs, it is probably time to shop around for someone new.

> Her solution to every problem is a prescription.
Beware, beware! A doctor who writes out a prescription within minutes of your visit may be trying to cover up your symptoms that may be treated without drugs. Is your doctor hiding behind a prescription pad? Sometimes, you may simply need more time to be understood, not just to be told, "If this drug doesn't work, I'll give you something else." According to the National Council of Patient Information and Education, over 80 percent of visits involved medication therapy in 1998; 36.5 percent of patients received two or more prescriptions; over 10 percent received four or more prescriptions.[4] Moreover, a majority of the top ten prescription medicines, ranked in order by 1999 retail sales, were: Prilosec, Lipitor, Prozac, Prevacid, Zocor, Zoloft, Claritin, Paxil, Norvasc and Augmentin. As a recovering prescription addict, it is important for you to avoid treating minor symptoms such as runny nose, congestion, headache or sore muscles with drugs. Tell your doctor to explain your diagnosis and then take part in decisions concerning your health, rather than masking symptoms with drugs. If your disorder is bearable and not a life threatening condition, as an addict, don't put yourself at risk of relapse if at all possible.

> He "tells me" what I'm going to do.
Some doctors leave you with an impression of: "We do things my way, or I won't see you again." Such doctors get irritated when patients voice an opinion about health decisions, considering this a sign of disrespect. Patient and doctor should have a mutual respect for one another. Any healthcare provider who does not appreciate that it's your life and your quality of life at

stake should be replaced. Your healthcare should constitute a partnership involving communication, decision-making and follow-up that will lead to a better prognosis for you and a healthy physician-patient relationship.

The idea of dropping your current doctor and looking for someone new may seem like an overwhelming task. But it doesn't have to be. Don't let changing doctors become a stressful affair. Following are some tips on how to change healthcare providers without anxiety.

First, choosing a new doctor will take some research on your part. A recommendation from a patient who has varied experience with a doctor is a good start. Also, if you know some unbiased healthcare workers who have worked with a variety of doctors, ask them. Their recommendations could be valuable. Sometimes local publications run lists of doctors most recommended by other healthcare workers in their fields. Also, it is especially important that you find a physician knowledgeable about addictive medications, for this will be a key step in safeguarding both your health and sobriety. Such a physician can help a recovering addict weigh possible alternatives to popping pills for minor pain, anxiety or sleeplessness. Recovered members of your support group may give you information about who to choose and who to avoid based on this special criterion. Make a list of doctors based on the recommendations you've received and check to see which physicians are members of your healthcare insurance plan. Be sure to remove from your list all the names of those doctors whose services will not be covered by your health insurance.

Once you have narrowed your list of recommended physicians, interview several before you leave the old one. Doctors who won't agree to an introductory interview are ones you probably shouldn't consider. Some professionals will charge a nominal fee for a fifteen-minute visit, but most doctors will not charge anything. Determine the charging policy up front on the phone.

After you have chosen your new doctor, his/her office staff will help you arrange to have records and lab reports forwarded from your former doctor. Your new doctor will need your signature giving authority to request copies of your records from your former doctor. Also, check with your managed-care plan about changing doctors as some have rules about how often you can switch doctors.

You don't need to make excuses to your original doctor. It's not necessary to explain anything to your former doctor, especially if you think you may return to him or her. However, if your previous doctor's behavior was disrespectful or inappropriate, consider writing to tell him or her why you're leaving. HMO and PPO plans are also interested in your grievance about any doctor they represent. It's in their best interest to pay attention to any letters of dissatisfaction, so they won't refer other patients to unsatisfactory doctors or even include them in their plan. Medical State Board investigators are increasingly pursuing disciplinary investigations of doctors who behave inappropriately, so serious misconduct should be reported to your state regulatory agency.

When you make your first visit after selecting your new physician, honestly and openly explain your addiction disease and your concerns about relapse. Once your new doctor is made aware of your history with addiction, the two of you can work together to lessen the risk of relapse with prescribed and non-prescribed medicines.

Always ask the doctor what your diagnosis is before a new prescription is written. Do not ask for or accept a prescription written for tolerable, passing symptoms.

When a prescription is written, ask why the medication is being prescribed, how to use it correctly and what side effects may be experienced.

Make and keep a follow-up appointment with the doctor when the medication is finished.

Though it sounds relatively simple on paper, finding a new doctor will take some work and some time. Again, it does not need to be a stressful or anxiety-inducing task. Do not let fear of dealing with this problem prevent you from seeking a new primary care physician; this task is essential if your current doctor aided—knowingly or unknowingly—your addiction to prescription medication. Remember the first four steps so necessary in battling addiction: finding a treatment center, obtaining a therapist, joining a support group and getting a sponsor. Don't hesitate to rely on the aid of one or all of these four resources if you need support or assistance when seeking a new doctor.

$$>>>5$$

DIAGNOSIS:
"When I finally got clean,
I discovered I was still sick."

When you arrive—high, woozy and disoriented—at a hospital, treatment center or physician, diagnosis may seem like a no-brainer: You are an addict. The arsenal of pills in your purse or pocket and the drugs in your bloodstream will tell the doctors to what you are addicted. The initial treatment is fairly clear: Get you off drugs; detox your system.

After that, the picture gets muddled, because addiction is not only a physical and biological affliction, but also a complex behavior pattern with varying causes and manifestations. You have to alleviate the symptoms and at the same time address the causes. Addiction is rarely simple. Up to 75 percent of people in drug treatment centers have what is known as **cross-addiction**, that is, a dependence on more than one drug or chemical. Moreover, national mental health sources suggest that up to 70 percent of people addicted to mood-altering chemicals have a **dual diagnosis**, that is, another mental illness along with addiction.

We who are addicted don't come into treatment saying, "I am addicted to several substances and behaviors," nor do we say, "I am an addict, but I have a dual diagnosis, so let's explore my other mental problems, too." We don't blurt out all our behaviors and problems, because we are either afraid to reveal too much or we are ignorant ourselves of all that is troubling us.

Therefore, the diagnosing physician or team must know how to discover all the addict's significant disorders with or without that person's cooperation. At the same time, the recovering prescription addict must learn how to live and cope with the complexities of his or her layered illnesses.

63

Cross-Addiction

In 1989, during her husband's unsuccessful presidential campaign, Kitty Dukakis checked into a private clinic in Newport, Rhode Island, for treatment for dependence on alcohol. The Massachusetts First Lady confessed much later in the campaign to a twenty-six-year addiction to amphetamine diet pills, a reliance she had overcome in 1982. Or thought she overcame. In reality, it appears that she gave up the amphetamine dependence for alcoholism.

Says counselor Fred Holmquist of the Hazelden Foundation in Center City, Minnesota, where Dukakis was treated for amphetamine abuse, cross-addiction is "like switching staterooms on the Titanic."[1]

While Dukakis and millions of others have gone from taking one legal drug to another, many people are dependent on several mood-altering substances at the same time. In another famous case of cross-addiction, former First Lady Betty Ford mixed liquor and tranquilizers. Her experience with addiction and recovery led her to found the famous Betty Ford Clinic in Rancho Mirage, California. When you read about celebrities going into treatment, you often hear they have been abusing several substances.

However, it can be dangerous to cite celebrity examples of drug addiction, because it may lead people to believe that the pressures of fame, the wild life of Hollywood and the medical gurus of exotic drugs in Tinseltown create a special situation where addiction is able to happen. The next logical step is to assume addiction can't happen to "ordinary" people like you and me.

As an "ordinary" person, I can tell you that you may quickly become addicted to several drugs as soon as you are addicted to the first one. After becoming hooked on one drug, for the addict seeking mood alteration, almost any other drug will do in a pinch. When I went into treatment, I had thirty-seven pills in my purse of probably a dozen different kinds. Almost any pill would do for me, because if I took enough, almost any medication, even over-the-counter medicine, would give me a buzz or a black-out, thus saving me from the necessity of dealing with the real world.

I've heard many stories from recovering addicts citing the use of several drugs together or switching from one to another. They didn't realize their behavior would lead to addiction, let alone abuse of a variety of drugs. This lack of initial intention is one thing that distinguishes prescription addiction from addiction to illegal drugs.

One recovering prescription addict remembers that when she was first admitted into treatment, she told her therapist she was addicted to her painkillers.

I'd had back surgery and was given painkillers for pain. The doctor told me to take them "as needed" (written on the prescription as prn), so I did without question or hesitation. I quickly got addicted and needed help. I went into a treatment program for two weeks until I felt well enough to go home. When I got home I felt good, but I couldn't sleep through the night. The next day I went to the store and bought over-the-counter sleeping aids, never realizing that I couldn't or shouldn't have them. I didn't know I could relapse with them. I took them every night, not realizing at first that I was addicted. All I knew was they were helping me sleep. After a month I decided to not take anymore and I discovered I couldn't sleep. So I continued my new habit.

My therapist noticed a mood change in me and asked about the prescriptions that I'd been on lately. I proudly told her I was only taking the prescribed medications and not abusing them as I had before. Then she asked me about over-the-counter medicines. I told her I had been taking sleeping aids, because I thought they were safe. I figured since anyone could buy them, they couldn't possibly be addictive. I was wrong. I had to be readmitted into the treatment center for addiction. No one ever told me about the dangers of cross-addictions before.

Cross-addiction includes abuse not only of multiple substances, but of activities as well.

Gary, a recovering prescription addict, told his support group that when he became drug free, he felt as if something had died inside of him.

I honestly thought that if I gambled a little I would put excitement back in my life. I never put it together that pill addiction and gambling were the same. I started out playing dollar numbers on the Lottery, which eventually lead to one-hundred-dollar-a-day numbers. My checks began to bounce, my credit cards were maxed and I borrowed from family and friends. When my wife found out, she was furious. My sister rescued me and helped me locate Gamblers Anonymous.

Gary's story illustrates the fact that kicking one addiction leaves a void, which must be filled. According to Dr. Robert Lefever, director of Promise Recovery Centre in London, "Cross-addiction is the inevitable outcome of treating individual addictions without tackling the root cause—inner loneliness."

If the root cause is not eliminated through therapy, other addictive behaviors may replace or accompany substance abuse. Common addictions are gambling and eating disorders, but doing anything to excess or to the point that it is detrimental to you or your family is considered addictive behavior. This might include excessive television watching, computer game playing or on-line chatting—activities that are not harmful in appropriate amounts. Addictive behavior might also include excessive participation in sexual activity, exercise and work—normally healthy activities in the appropriate contexts, but unhealthy when used inappropriately or in excess to avoid dealing with boredom, tension, stress, fatigue, pressure and loneliness.

My cross-addiction was shopping. I bought things I didn't need. I bought things I didn't remember buying. I bought things I couldn't afford. I started out doing it unconsciously; I just thought I deserved something new for myself. The euphoric feeling I felt when I bought something, no matter how short a time it lasted, gave me a sense of inner peace and pleasure. What I didn't realize was that I had a cross-addiction and it was excessive shopping.

Here's how it happened. Shortly after coming home from my treatment center, no longer filled with pills and alcohol, I was so proud of myself I thought I deserved a reward (and my husband agreed). I chose the reward carefully, deciding to buy myself a new sweater. I couldn't wait to get up, dress and go out to the car, all the while thinking about where to shop, which mall to visit first. I was so excited, I felt as if I was high again on pills. My legs couldn't walk fast enough in and out of all the stores filled with pretty clothes and shoes. By the end of the day, I not only found my perfect sweater, but also picked out slacks, shoes, a purse, a blouse and jewelry to match. My husband never saw the bill, because I hid it from him just as I once had hidden my pills. I only showed him my sweater since that's what I told him I was buying. Later, my euphoric feelings were quickly replaced by shame and embarrassment. I was amazed I could lie so easily. The habit of deceit I had developed over the years to hide my drug addiction had taken over once again. I somehow justified my behavior by telling myself that at least I wasn't still taking prescription pills, never recognizing my compulsive shopping as a new addiction. I continued my second bad habit for almost a year before my hefty credit card bills and bounced checks caught up with me. I dreaded telling my husband, but I had to before the phone calls from creditors started. After I promised I would talk to my counselor and sponsor about this new abuse, my husband took my credit cards and checkbook away until we could get the bills lowered.

It was only in therapy that I recognized my shopping "problem" also was an addiction. It was not a new addiction, but the same old addiction in a new guise. Another inanimate object had replaced my pills and had become my new best friend. I had found something else to preoccupy my mind. I found it easier to cover up my emotional pain by spending money rather than talking about the pain and working through it. I still had not come to grips with my feelings or living in the "real world." I thought I could work on my treatment and still have an escape without paying the consequences.

For prescription addicts, the most common cross-addiction is abuse of alcohol, but there are other significant areas of abuse as well.

Alcohol Abuse: A healthy person knows when to stop drinking alcohol and sets limits prior to drinking. When he or she reaches that limit—whether it's a certain number of drinks or a certain feeling, the in-control person stops. The addict does not. Those who are alcoholics convince themselves that they need alcohol because they're shy or because it calms their anxiety or anger. If they have used alcohol before, it seems natural to do it again, even while taking prescription drugs.

Kerri, a recovering prescription addict says, "I used alcohol with my pills to speed up the effects, not realizing that I could pass out or die after a few drinks."

Statistics show that women are more likely than men to use alcohol in conjunction with pills. The varied reasons include that some women don't listen to their doctors' warnings about drinking while taking prescribed drugs or their doctors don't warn them of the dangers of mixing the two substances. Statistics show that 90 percent of drug overdoses involve women who are abusing legal substances, such as alcohol or prescription drugs. Alcohol is the most common second drug chosen by the prescription addict.

Gambling: All types of gambling can become addictive, regardless of whether a person gambles on races, games, numbers or plays with tickets, machines or cards. According to the National Gambling Impact Study Commission Act, in 1995 approximately $500 billion was wagered in the United States. According to that report, 70 percent of the United States adult population had gambled in the past year. Sooner or later, virtually all compulsive gamblers resort to illegal activities to support their gambling addiction. After all, money is the substance of their addiction. German researcher Gerhard Meyer in a recent issue of *Biological Psychiatry* noted that "Physiological responses to gambling enhance mood and...winning has the ability to produce a euphoric state." In Meyer's study, ten men played blackjack at a casino. When playing for money, the men's heart rates and hormonal secretions rose considerably more than when they didn't play for money. The release of hormones when betting produces a rush similar to that of certain drugs and may be just as addictive.[2] The risk itself is exciting and the lure of the big prize on the next ticket or roll of the dice is reinforced by occasional pay-offs. Almost all gambling opportunities, including state-run lotteries, are advertised with a heavy emphasis on the big win; none mention, at least not loudly or in large print, the constant risk and the unrelenting losses of players. Those on the borderline between rational judgment and the desire for an emotional lift may be pulled over the edge into gambling.

Sex: According to Patrick Carnes, director of sexual disorders at the Arizona Treatment Center, a growing number of executives and professionals—lawyers, doctors, bankers, brokers and CEOs—are risking their careers and families for sex, whether for affection, physical thrills or control.[3] Individuals in all walks of life who are addicted to sex risk losing their marriages, families, jobs and reputations, not to mention contracting diseases that could kill them. Men and women addicted to sex believe they can flout the rules and remain immune to consequences. The majority of sex addicts describe their families of origin as emotionally detached, rigid and frequently with one or both parents fighting their own addictions. Emotionally, these individuals never grew up. As adults, they may be super-conscientious on the job, but psychologically, they're impaired. They have a lot of anger and anxiety. Many of them are depressed and don't know it. The only thing most of them do know is that they feel unlovable.

Carnes sees many cross-addictions among sex addicts. According to him, many will first get high on their drug of choice—pills, alcohol and/or narcotics—to get rid of their inhibitions. Then, there's the conquest. Later, they frequently feel scared and embarrassed.

Karen, a recovering prescription addict, is a case in point.

I never thought my sexual behavior was a problem. I was competing in a mostly male corporate office. I thought about sex all the time, fantasizing about my co-workers. Then I cruised the bars and picked up men everywhere. I thought it validated me as a desirable woman. I came close to totally self-destructing. I never considered myself a sex addict until I entered treatment, but sex really is another kind of drug.

Eating disorders: Clinical Director Leonard Levitz of the Renfrew Center, a Philadelphia treatment center for eating disorders, found that many of the same factors that make people susceptible to other addictions also make them prone to eating disorders.[4]

A compulsive overeater centers her life around food the same way an alcoholic does with alcohol. Food acts as a tranquilizer. These people will eat a box of cookies or an entire cake to make themselves feel good or as a way to relieve stress. Cravings for sweets may also be linked to the same physiological mechanism that sets up an addiction to drugs. Recovering alcoholics have often noted a craving for sweets.

The opposite behavior, but the same addictive process, is apparent in anorexia. Charlotte explains what happened to her when she was in recovery.

I have always had a need to be in control of everything in my life. After undergoing treatment to understand all there was to understand about addiction, I still felt out of control for some reason. I thought everyone was controlling me—colleagues, friends and family. Then I got the bright idea that the one thing no one but me could control was how I ate. So I ate one meal a day or none at all, just snacks. I lost twenty pounds in six weeks. Eventually I realized this was another cross-addiction I needed to learn about and learn to live with.

For some, the addiction starts with dieting. When stress and guilt over her troubled marriage came to the forefront, Carolyn began to lose weight. She got down to a size two. At the time, she never considered herself an addict. After all, Carolyn didn't take pills and she wasn't much of a drinker. However, she now realizes she was addicted to starving herself.

It took all of my concentration to avoid eating. You wouldn't think so, but it did. It kept my mind off what was really bothering me—a problem I couldn't cope with in my marriage.

Carolyn's mother and sister worried about her weight and her tiny appetite. They took her on a vacation. When she got up in the middle of the night to go for her third jog in twenty-four hours, they'd seen enough. In the morning they insisted she go to a doctor, who diagnosed her illness as anorexia. Luckily, Carolyn allowed herself to be cared for by the doctor, a nutritionist and a therapist who specialized in eating disorders. As she began to understand her disease, she slowly increased her eating, limited her running to reasonable hours, began to change her image of herself—and began drinking to excess. If she couldn't starve herself, she had to do something to ease the pain of things going wrong in her marriage. Now, still in the care of a therapist, she has turned to a healthier approach to dealing with her life—facing her problems using new insight and new skills. She has a long way to go because the pressures are great, but at least Carolyn is not adding illness to illness and crisis to crisis by altering her moods chemically or starving herself.

Other prescription addicts report gaining weight. One prescription addict confessed to weight gain of eighty pounds along with lack of interest in personal appearance. Compulsive overeating often accompanies or follows addiction to prescription drugs. Food brings comfort to those who feel guilty about their addiction or are just plain lost and lonely.

The habits just described—alcohol abuse, gambling, sex addiction and eating disorders—are some of the most problematic cross-addictions, but they do not comprise an all-inclusive list. Any substance or activity improperly used can become a dangerous addiction. Nicotine is an obviously addictive substance, as are coffee and other caffeinated products. People who drink coffee and smoke at the same time are using mild uppers and downers; likewise people who smoke while drinking alcohol are using two kinds of mood altering substances. Some habits are more problematic than others.

Even "virtuous" activities such as exercise and work can be addictions or cross-addictions. Ron was a runner. Like Carolyn, he ran miles and miles in all kinds of weather, becoming very skinny, because he didn't consume enough calories to compensate for those he lost running. His muscles looked great; his body fat composition was the envy of his friends, but he was not well. Ron ran to avoid thinking of a number of severe disappointments in his life. The admiration of his friends made up somewhat for his other seeming failures.

Then there's the workaholic. Jack worked seven days a week, fourteen hours a day. He enjoyed the amazement and admiration of his colleagues, but most of all he was working to the point of exhaustion so he wouldn't have to deal with discord with his wife or a lack of connectedness with his children. Whenever Jack's wife said anything that sounded like a complaint or a conflict in the making—during his brief waking periods at home—his hand automatically reached for his car keys. He would go to work. Day or night, he would remember something he needed to do at the office. No one could ever call his behavior anything but a virtue, Jack told himself. He was doing it all for his wife and children.

Work and exercise addictions often accompany substance abuse. One prescription addict tells how he always took a lot of pride and joy in providing a good lifestyle for his family.

Making my family proud and happy has always been a priority for me. After all, I was the "breadwinner" and I felt that was my role in life. I continually brought home a steady paycheck by working forty to forty-five hours a week. When I was popping pills, I probably took off an average of ten to fifteen hours a week between doctor shopping and going to different pharmacies so I wouldn't be labeled a "regular customer" at any one place.

After working with my addictionologist and psychiatrist to taper down my pills and eventually get off all unnecessary prescriptions and over-the-counter medicines, I vowed to take better care of myself and appreciate my family and their needs. One way to do this I thought was to make more money and give them more things to make them proud of me. My work always gave me pleasure, so I chose to increase my time at work to sixty to seventy hours a week.

What I called fun my family called being a workaholic. I thought if they saw me working hard, buying them new things and taking fewer vacations that I was doing good. My illness had transformed but not disappeared. Now I was getting high from working long hours and making lots of money. I admit it got me excited to see the extra money in our account, but my family questioned my motives. Was I helping them or was this just another way to avoid working on the underlying issues that had caused my prescription addiction? I discovered in therapy that I was covering up childhood and family issues. My father rarely was home. His work behavior told his kids that it was more important to provide a living than to provide a loving home. I remember being angry that I didn't have a father growing up, because we rarely saw him. I had to learn to balance my adult life so my wife, my children and I could all come out winners.

Addiction drives us to do things that are against our better judgment and are ultimately destructive in their consequences. The addict denies the addiction. The addict finds that the activity, situation or substance craved alters his mood in a desirable direction—in a way no other alternative can. Thus the habit grows into an addiction and becomes a "trusted friend" and, when the addiction ceases, the person feels he has lost his best friend. He's understandably anxious to find a replacement. The result: cross-addiction.

Dual Diagnosis

While I was in treatment, I was diagnosed with having multiple disorders: addiction to prescription drugs plus severe depression and post-traumatic stress syndrome. If I didn't believe the diagnosis then, I believed it after I became clean, because, instead of feeling happy, healthy and confident, I felt sad, empty, helpless and even suicidal. If this was sobriety, I didn't want it. I needed to come to grips with my "dual diagnosis," that is, the recognition of one or more mental disorders along with addiction. Ideally, diagnosis drives treatment. I was fortunate to be treated for both my addiction and my mental illnesses concurrently.

Dual diagnosis is not uncommon. Seven percent of the general population, that is, between fifteen and twenty million Americans, fall into the dual diagnosis category, suffering from both an addiction and a psychiatric illness. National mental health resources suggest that 50 percent to 70 percent of those who are addicted to mood altering chemicals also suffer from psychiatric disorders. Chemical dependency is found in 56 percent of people with bipolar disorder (manic depression), 47 percent of people with schizophrenia, 32 percent of people living with mood disorders other than bipolar and 24 percent of people with anxiety disorder.

People who have one disorder are obviously at higher risk for developing related disorders. For example, an individual may have two disorders, each of which represents an alternative response to a similar set of problems or one disorder leads to the development of another.

The American Psychiatric Association in Washington, D.C. has published a list of the mental illnesses most commonly linked with substance abuse in a Fourth Edition of the *Diagnostic and Statistical Manual of Mental Disorders*.[5] They are:

> *Antisocial personality disorder*: A pervasive pattern of disregard for, and violation of, the rights of others. The disorder is characterized in part by risk-taking, criminality and pathological lying.
> *Anxiety disorders*: A group of disorders characterized by unrealistic fear, panic or avoidance behavior. These disorders include (among others) panic attacks, phobias, obsessive-compulsive disorder and generalized anxiety disorder.
> *Bipolar disorder*: A disorder characterized by alternating manic and depressive episodes.
> *Depressive disorders*: A group of disorders including various forms of depression and manic-depression.
> *Generalized anxiety disorder*: A disorder characterized by at least six months of persistent and excessive anxiety and worry not resulting from exposure to a drug or medication.
> *Major depressive episode*: A period of at least two weeks during

which there is either depressed mood or the loss of interest or pleasure in nearly all activities.
> *Mania*: A period of abnormally and persistently elevated, expansive
  or irritable mood.
> *Mood disorders*: Depressive and manic disorders.
> *Panic disorders*: A disorder characterized by sudden, unexpected and
  persistent episodes of intense fear, accompanied by a sense of immi-
  nent danger and an urge to escape.
> *Phobia*: A marked and persistent fear of a specific object or situation
  not normally feared.
> *Post-traumatic Stress disorder*: A disorder often brought on by major
  emotional trauma such as sexual or physical assault. It is characterized
  by the re-experiencing of the traumatic event (in dreams, illusions or
  hallucinations) and by avoidance of stimuli associated with the trauma.
> *Schizophrenia*: A chronic disorder characterized by illusions, halluci-
  nations and disorganized thoughts and behaviors.

The American Board of Psychiatry and the American Society of Addiction
Medicine states, "It is critical to identify the coexistence of a major psychiatric
disorder or personality disorder because if it is not appropriately treated, it
often results in relapse to substance abuse. To complicate matters, individuals
may present with various types of psychiatric symptoms as a result of their
response and reaction to involvement with addiction treatment."[6]

The combination of depression and addiction often causes diagnostic
difficulty for healthcare providers trying to determine appropriate treatment. According to Steven Lynn, M.D., depression and addiction have much
in common.[7] The medical community considers both depression and addictive disorders to be biological, psychological and social illnesses. Prescription
addiction can masquerade as depression or manic depression, so the distinction must be made between depressive symptoms that are a part of
addiction or withdrawal and depressive illness itself. This is made difficult by
the similarities: impulsiveness, difficulty concentrating and feelings of hope-
lessness, helplessness, inferiority and grandiosity. And, of course, denial.

When a dual diagnosis is made correctly, treatment can be individualized
more effectively. Unfortunately, many people don't know they have dual disorders until treatment has already begun. Their healthcare providers may
make a belated dual diagnosis or the patients may discover a second disorder
on their own through another mishap in their life, such as ongoing depression
or compulsion to abuse another addiction.

"I felt I didn't fall into any category for treatment until I began to read books on dual diagnosis," says Erin, another recovered addict. "Then I found a therapist who understood prescription addiction and depression occurring together, so that I didn't need to find two different doctors to treat each illness."

The prognosis is much poorer when a misdiagnosis is made and carried forward. This is what happened to Tony, now a recovered addict.

When I first began treatment with my therapist I thought I was being treated for prescription addiction only. I didn't feel depressed, but my moods were like a roller coaster out of control. I thought I was just hyperactive, because that was what doctors told my parents years ago. They prescribed Ritalin. I quickly got addicted to it, even sold it to other kids as speed. After two or three visits with my current therapist, she told me I had been misdiagnosed and that I wasn't hyperactive but bipolar, meaning I had extreme mood swings (highs and lows). I felt angry about the earlier misdiagnosis, but was glad that I now have the answers to my nightmare.

The difference between addiction alone and dual diagnosis is illustrated by Carol and Shawna, whose stories have been related in previous chapters. Carol was afraid to tell her husband she had been addicted to painkillers throughout their entire marriage. She wanted desperately to quit, but she was sure he would be very judgmental and perhaps even divorce her. So she worked it out with her doctor to supervise her withdrawal and recovery at home without her husband ever knowing. She has been sober now for two years. To this day, her husband is unaware of her condition. Carol characterized herself before addiction as strong and clearheaded. It appears she became addicted to painkillers after surgery without suffering from depression or any other mental disorder throughout. Her recovery wasn't easy, but it was possible without inpatient treatment, frequent relapses or emotional breakdown. In contrast to this, Shawna, who during her youth had twenty-some unnecessary surgeries just to obtain legally prescribed painkillers, suffered depression and even suicidal thoughts for decades. Now recovered, she often logs on to prescription addiction Web sites on the Internet to offer support and encouragement to addicts who tell their stories on-line. When someone desperate to escape addiction says he plans to do it at home or asks if it's possible to do it at home, Shawna tells them resoundingly, "NO. I've tried it numerous times and it doesn't work." She is speaking as an addict with a dual diagnosis and she speaks the truth as she knows it. Recovery at home is extremely difficult for any addict and it is virtually impossible for those with other mental disorders—dual diagnoses as yet undiagnosed.

Why do some people have dual diagnoses?

1. Some individuals may have a mental illness that creates feelings of sadness, anxiety or fear and then turn to prescription drugs or alcohol for relief, creating a whole new set of problems.
2. Some may start with addiction to prescription medication or other substances that alter brain chemistry and other organs. As the drug assaults normal brain function, mental illness may develop as a result.
3. Others may have both disorders at the same time and independently; one illness does not cause the other, but it can affect the other.

Many counselors who work with dual-disorder clients are often distracted by the "chicken or the egg" question. That is, did the prescription medication addiction come first or did the psychiatric disorder? It doesn't matter! In either case, the risk of relapse is high if therapy doesn't recognize and address both conditions effectively. Treatment is hampered when the medical professionals who treat the mental illness and those who treat the addiction are not working in concert.

Treatment

Whatever its origin, the pain and suffering caused by mental illness is just as real as that caused by a physical illness. Mental health practitioners work with patients to first alleviate the pain, then treat the underlying causes of the problem. Treatment may consist of medication, individual counseling/therapy, group therapy and family counseling/therapy. It may involve an inpatient hospitalization (treatment facility), partial hospitalization or intensive or regular outpatient treatment. In any case, there are several serious issues unique to dual diagnosis that must be dealt with at each stage of treatment.

According to the Department of Health and Human Services' Center for Substance Abuse Prevention, there are three effective approaches to treating dual disorders:

1. **Sequential treatment:** The person goes first to one kind of therapy and then to the other, alternating procedures.
2. **Parallel treatment:** A person participates in two different kinds of treatment at the same time.
3. **Integrated treatment:** Generally the most effective, in this plan the individual gets help for both disorders in one treatment program.[8]

In integrated treatment, an addicted individual with a co-occurring disorder stands a better chance of being in the care of a professional who understands both problems and who is willing to address the special challenges of a dual diagnosis. Integrated treatment strives to provide clients with the necessary tools to cope with stressful situations, to improve their ability to get along in daily life and to help them make positive changes toward a healthy lifestyle.

The American Psychiatric Association says that, ideally, dual diagnosis requires special training of the treatment team members in both chemical dependency programs and psychiatric programs. This is especially important because the typical treatments for each have some major differences with which the treatment team must be familiar.

Typical Treatments for Addiction and Psychiatric Disorders

Psychiatric Treatment	Addiction Treatment
1. Goal: Resolution of mental disorder or symptom relief.	1. Goal: Recovery; Stabilize sobriety
2. Use medication as needed	2. Abstinence: Avoid medications except for those closely supervised by healthcare professionals.
3. Psychiatrist writes orders and informs staff.	3. Treatment decisions made by a team. No quick changes and attention paid to enabling and splitting behaviors.
4. Program flexible: Emphasis on communication, relationships and decision-making skills.	4. Program structured: Emphasis on active learning, support meetings and family involvement.
5. Discharge when symptoms are under control with psychotherapy and/or psychotropic drug therapy.	5. Discharge when patient develops and demonstrates ability to work his/her personal recovery plan.

Professionals trained in one setting often have difficulty adapting to or accepting the differences in other treatment approaches. It is imperative to seek treatment from healthcare professionals who are comfortable with the differing demands of the coexisting disorders in dual diagnosis.

Another treatment issue is insurance coverage. Some health insurance packages do cover both substance abuse and mental health problems—dual diagnoses—but caregivers often are forced to modify treatment to meet strict insurance guidelines. Todd Barlow, Director of Drug and Alcohol services at Penn Foundation in Sellerville, Pennsylvania, says most insurance companies cover dual diagnoses, but "ask caregivers to treat patients for one or the other (illness), not both at the same time.

"First a person gets their addiction problem treated and, once they're stabilized, they get mental health treatment," Barlow says. "This can't work. It's the reason for the phrase dual diagnosis—the two are interactive. A person is clean for three months and then the insurance company says go ahead and switch to mental health treatment, but not everything fits into that neat little box."[9] Because each part of a dual disorder can aggravate the course of the other, both disorders must be treated together to have the best chance for a positive outcome.

In dual diagnosis cases, extra and special education must be given to the recovering patient. According to Nancy Conover, clinical supervisor at Hyland Psychiatric Center at St. Anthony's Medical Center in St. Louis, "Patients with dual illnesses need substantial education concerning their medication needs, a particularly challenging situation in these cases. Because recovery from chemical dependency requires abstinence from mood-altering chemicals, many chemically dependent patients have a difficult time accepting medication therapy as an aspect of their psychiatric treatment. It's crucial to help them realize the importance and necessity of their medication and how it must complement their therapy and recovery program components. A patient with a dual diagnosis can relapse just as easily by getting off the medication necessary to treat his or her psychiatric disorder as a chemically dependent individual can relapse by going back to active drinking or drug abuse."[10]

The duality of diagnosis and treatment must also be addressed in support groups. Chemical dependency support groups sometimes exclude recovering addicts who take medications for a mental illness. These groups, understandably wary of any and all addictive drugs, believe that any medication interferes with or precludes recovery by definition; they consider the use of any medication as a relapse. They lack the knowledge of psychiatric therapy necessary to evaluate and supervise people using prescription drugs. Among support groups, Prescription Anonymous recognizes dual diagnosis and teaches the recovering prescription addict how to live with the complexities of dual diagnosis and cross-addiction.

The single diagnosis of addiction can be difficult enough, but for those who have dual diagnosis, life can be even more frustrating and painful. It takes time to sort things out and a lot of patience to understand everything that's going on. Some may have difficulty holding onto a job, living independently or developing satisfying relationships. Relapse is a constant risk. Thoughts of suicide as a way out are never totally absent from the mind.

Dual disorders can affect virtually any area of family functioning as well, including the mood and atmosphere in homes, roles assumed by family members, rules by which the family operates, relationships and communication among members, cohesion and the ability to confront and solve problems. Moreover, legal problems, the high risk of incarceration, work problems and higher incidents of emergency room visits, as well as multiple admissions for psychiatric care, chemical dependency services and acute healthcare take a toll on addicted individuals' and family members' patience and financial resources.

The good news, however, is that recognizing mental illnesses that accompany addiction and treating the dual diagnosis appropriately give the doubly afflicted prescription addict about the same chance of recovery as his singly afflicted counterpart. Stop now and consider your own mental health. Ask your therapist to evaluate you thoroughly for additional mental disorders. You can overcome dual diagnosis. I have, Shawna did and many do every year. You can, too, now that you know that prescription addiction does not always attack alone. Knowledge is power.

THE FIRST THIRTY DAYS:

"I'm ready, but scared.
What can I expect?"

The necessary decision for beginning day one of recovery is found in your heart and mind. Recovery is possible if you want it badly enough. Admitting to yourself or someone else that you have become powerless over your addiction and that you need help is a good beginning.

But making the decision to get help in a treatment facility, hospital, clinic or even on your own can be frightening. Your heart is troubled with self-doubt and your mind is racing with questions such as the ones below, which prescription addicts often ask themselves.

1. What's going to happen to me physically and mentally without my pills or other mood-altering substances?
In the case of addiction recovery, fear of the unknown is more debilitating than fear of the known. The truth about withdrawal from addictive substances is daunting, but you will be tougher if you know what to expect. Physical symptoms vary; the longer you have been abusing and misusing prescription drugs, the longer and more severe the symptoms you may experience. Detoxification, better known as withdrawal, can last from four to seven days in its acute form. You can experience chills, sweats, nausea, vomiting, shakiness, anxiety, fatigue, restlessness, headache, muscle pain, seizures, depression and rage. Lesser symptoms can last for weeks or even months. Depression, varying in degrees from mild to severe, is common and normal for most people going through withdrawal. Withdrawal from certain

chemicals, opiates, for example, can be deadly if done too quickly. In a treat-ment center, detoxing is done in a way that is safe for you. Also, some of the worst withdrawal symptoms can be somewhat alleviated with medication that does not contribute to your addiction. This is a definite advantage of detoxing in a treatment center versus on your own.

2. How can I stand the discomfort of withdrawal and how can I not give up?

Don't think, "Oh, I'm in this pain and suffering for days and I can't make it." Instead, think only about the next three minutes: "I'm in this pain and suf-fering for these three minutes. I can stand it for just three minutes." Then at two and three-quarters minutes, think, "I got through two and three-quar-ters minutes, so I can stand it for another couple of minutes." Keep on con-gratulating yourself on the few minutes you have lived through without pills and extend your goal to cover the next few minutes. Soon you can do this for hours instead of minutes. For every chunk of time that is behind you, you are closer to your goal of sobriety, responsibility and self-respect. If you give up and take some pills now, you will have to go through this same painful chunk of time again the next time you try to kick the habit and you don't want to do that. Remember the suffering, keep a journal, if you can, so that this mem-ory will serve as a deterrent to ever going back. You do not want to have to do this more than once.

3. How can I trust strangers in a treatment facility enough to give them control over me?

A treatment facility gives you a safe environment to help improve your chances for success. It removes you from all outside pressures and triggers associated with the bad habits that you now have. A treatment facility or clinic gives you a "time out" from the outside world until you are strong enough to face it alone. This could last anywhere from seven to twenty-five days. Live-in programs available for further support and continued supervi-sion and monitoring of behaviors may allow you as long as six to nine months. The patient and therapist together make the final decision for the best treatment plan.

Trusting strangers at a treatment facility can be hard at first, because addicts usually have not trusted others for a long time, instead choosing to isolate themselves from family, friends, co-workers and marriage partners for months, perhaps years. Staff counselors are sensitive to issues of trust and are trained to help patients cope and adjust to this difficult time in their lives. They are usually very kind, patient people who show empathy and sincerity. They can help you talk through your options and can answer every question you have regarding the facility and the level of care that you will receive there. Trusting people doesn't usually happen overnight, but it does and can happen, gradually, at your own pace and in your own time.

4. I'm too embarrassed and ashamed to show my weakness, stupidity or illness to anyone. I haven't shown anyone my real self in months, maybe years. How can I do it now?
When I was admitted into the treatment facility, I was embarrassed, rebellious and angry because I felt that I was smarter than other addicts were. After all, I felt I knew better than they did not to abuse or misuse my prescription drugs. I somehow had just gotten caught up in prescription addiction and now I had this tenacious disease to deal with. I was angry. Later I learned that other prescription addicts feel similarly and some feel worse. After covering up addictions for so long, most recovering addicts aren't sure who they are anymore. It takes days for some, weeks for others, to begin to shed their feelings of anger, weakness, stupidity and embarrassment. You have to try very hard not to believe that you're a bad person for being biologically vulnerable to this disease. Family, friends and marriages do heal from such an upheaval and people do forgive. Your efforts will pay off in the long run. Life can be good again if you want it strongly enough. My therapist tells me that I am my own worst critic and extremely hard on myself, as are most addicts. I can forgive everyone else but myself, I hear many addicts say. Discovering and achieving recovery makes us the smartest, strongest and sincerest people.

5. The thought of explaining my disease to my unsuspecting spouse, family or children breaks my heart and might break theirs, too. How can I deal with that?
My own way of life while an addict consisted of manipulating, lying and stealing from people to maintain my secret habit. It included hiding my prescription addiction from my spouse, family, children and friends. This negative, secret lifestyle had become normal to me. This is not uncommon among those of us who have abused substances. Our spouses are often the last people to know; they often never suspect the fact that their wives or husbands could have such a disease. Some unsuspecting husbands and wives don't find out until they receive phone calls from therapists or hospitals telling them their spouses overdosed and were rushed to hospital emergency

rooms. In other cases, addicts have been able to break the news to their spouses, families and children at home or in another quiet meeting place. There they nervously tell their loved ones they have been abusing prescription drugs and confess that they need to get help.

Most prescription addicts are quite surprised and pleased with their loved ones' reactions. Family members often say they suspected there was a problem, but didn't know how to ask or approach the person about it. Many express relief to learn what the problem is and to know that their loved one is ready to get help. They usually offer to support the addicted person in any way. Nevertheless, some addicts have had loved ones who are taken by complete surprise and are quick to judge their addicted relative harshly, even accusing them of being dishonest and lying. Yet even when family members react negatively at first, they often become supportive later and offer help with recovery.

6. I'm scared and angry. What can I do about that?

I was very angry and scared when I realized that I was not in control of my own life. Pills that were once prescribed to me to improve my health, including those that I had misused from the pharmacy shelves, were now in control of me and that was a frightening realization. My sponsor and therapist told me to get my feelings out. They urged me not to carry the burden alone. Now I urge others to not be angry or scared alone. Millions of people have felt and feel the same way you do. Sharing with other prescription addicts, sponsor, therapist, friends, family and spiritual advisors can all help in recovery. Also, expressing yourself in a journal and physical activities like aerobics, sports, martial arts or walking provide a good release of emotion without harmful consequences.

7. Will I be cured of this disease?

Unfortunately, the disease of addiction afflicts millions of people who have inherited or acquired addictive personality traits that make it extremely dangerous for them to use any mood-altering substance ever again. Thus, they are never truly "cured" of the affliction. Together with support groups, sponsors and therapists to help monitor behavior and manage prescribed medications, recovered addicts can live as happy and healthy lives as other people, but must never forget the disease still lurks close by, ready to destroy their lives if they let it.

8. Does everybody have to go to a treatment facility? Can I go through withdrawal on my own?

Making the decision to go to a treatment facility, clinic or hospital can be a difficult one. This decision is best to make with the guidance of a family physician or therapist.

Treatment facilities are very thorough in their patient assessments which help determine exactly what the best treatment plan should be for you. The therapists, staff counselors, nurses and group therapy leaders together are able to monitor your progress to determine any need for changes in your treatment or medications.

Treatment center staff know what's best for you while in a crisis situation even if, at the moment, you don't agree or understand. Addicts have tried doing it "their way" with disastrous results, so we must have faith that specialized treatment facilities know what has worked with others and trust they can apply their wisdom to us.

Not everyone goes to a treatment facility, however. Some undergo the process of withdrawal with the strict supervision of their therapist, addictionologist or physician. These people gradually taper down the dosage of pills to minimize the physical withdrawal symptoms. Frequent follow-up visits allow professionals to monitor blood pressure and any side effects to treatment. Counseling helps with any psychological problems that need to be discussed.

Here again is a diagram showing advantages of receiving care at a treatment facility and the disadvantages of trying it on your own.

Advantages of a Treatment Facility

Medication management
Support groups
Safe environment
Detoxification supervised
Suicide watch
Non-judgmental environment
Vital signs monitored daily
Depression supervised
Not feeling isolated or alone
Changed behaviors learned

Disadvantages of Going Through Withdrawal at Home Without Professional Supervision

No supervision of withdrawal symptoms
Health risks
Depression and isolation
No guidance or support link
Anxiety
Dangerous environment (triggers)
Confusion and fear
Lack of self-esteem

---

9. **I've heard of Rapid Detox where you go to a hospital and in a couple days you're rid of the drugs. Isn't that a way to do it quickly without suffering or taking too many days off from work?**

Rapid Detox is a medical treatment for addiction to opiates only. Besides heroin and methadone, this family of drugs includes the prescription medication Lortab, Vicodin, Darvocet, Percocet, codeine and others. Going "cold turkey" from opiates without medical treatment can damage the cardio-pulmonary and the central nervous systems, so detoxing by conventional treatment has required days or weeks. Rapid Detox offers a new, quicker alternative by chemically reversing the effects of opiates in your brain which "require" an ever-increasing amount of the drugs. The procedure must be done in a closely supervised medical setting while the patient is under anesthesia for several (three to six) hours. The anesthesia prevents the patient from feeling the worst of his withdrawal symptoms.

Rapid Detox is not, however, "an easy way out." The patient will experience moderate withdrawal symptoms such as nausea, vomiting, muscle cramps and shaking for several hours after waking up and nervousness and insomnia for several weeks. It does not treat dual diagnosis at all, so symptoms of other mental disorders such as depression will persist. The most important thing you should know is that Rapid Detox in no way eliminates the need for a recovery program. Its success, like that of other treatment methods, depends on the patient's motivation and a full program of counseling and possibly medication therapy. Abstinence needs to be supported by peer groups, sponsors and understanding family members, just as absti-nence following any other withdrawal method. Do not have this treatment without a full recovery program in place. You will be wasting your money. Rapid Detox is sometimes, but not often, covered by health insurance. It currently costs from $4500 to $7500.

One treatment center featured on ABC News claimed for its Rapid Detox treatment a 50 percent success rate at one year post-treatment, verified when possible by urine tests after three months, six months and one year. A 50 percent success rate is about the same as the overall success rate for all other methods of withdrawal from prescription drugs.

In short, the program you use for withdrawal isn't the most important issue; it's the recovery program that keeps you off drugs.

10. If I detoxify at a treatment center, how long will I be there and what happens when I get out?

The therapist, staff counselors and the patient determine the number of days a person stays in a treatment facility. The average length of time is seven to ten days. If you're on suicide watch, it is a law in most states that patients be observed and not released in fewer than seventy-two hours. Your insurance policy may also determine how many days of inpatient treatment you will get. You will need to pay out-of-pocket if you want or need treatment beyond what your insurance will pay for.

Once you are detoxed and emotionally stable enough to be discharged, you will meet with staff counselors and your therapist to make plans for your continued care on an outpatient basis.

Some patients may choose to live in a halfway house, without locked doors or windows, where supervision and group therapy can be continued. Live-in programs have female and male residents who are supervised by house managers. The managers make sure the rules of the house are fol-lowed as well as provide residents with guidance in attending support groups and transportation to doctor appointments. Here patients in recov-ery learn to become independent yet able to ask for help when necessary and begin to get back into life with a new outlook. These programs deal with the physical, the emotional, the mental and the spiritual aspects of life. Many individuals greatly benefit from ongoing support in a stable, structured envi-ronment with other recovering people. It makes them feel less alone and they gain strength and knowledge from each other.

Discuss your after-treatment options with your therapist and family, but most importantly, be honest with yourself. Do you feel safe from the danger of abusing medications again? Are you emotionally stable enough to handle any other co-occurring illnesses?

When you do go home, your spouse or family members will also be counseled on how to best help you through the adjustment period. You will be particularly sensitive and insecure in the days, weeks and perhaps months after your discharge. Those around you need to learn to take care of themselves and not get too caught up in trying to "fix" your troubles, a behavior known as codependence. It's up to you to help yourself. Assuming this responsibility makes you stronger, healthier and happier.

Once at home, keep busy with support group meetings. Some people in recovery find it useful to go to meetings every day. Try not to be by yourself for long periods of time. Being alone can lead to feelings of depression, loneliness and temptation. The longer you stay in a program of recovery, the simpler life becomes as you learn and grow.

Recovery starts here. Making the decision to improve your quality of life by realizing your powerlessness over your addiction to prescription drugs and mood-altering chemicals is a gigantic step toward change. Putting yourself in the hands of professionals, far from imprisoning you, leaves you free to rebuild self-worth, self-esteem and self-confidence in a protective environment.

Shawna, a recovered prescription addict previously introduced, shares the thoughts and feelings she had during the first days of withdrawal. Her story reflects some of the attitudes and experiences as well as the feelings of desperation mixed with hope that we all have shared.

I was addicted to hydrocodone for over a decade and I overcame it. First of all, I didn't try to do it alone. I entered myself into a treatment center. When I detoxed, they told me what I was feeling (massive headaches, irritability, shakes, fear) was normal. If you taper down your pill intake, the withdrawal symptoms won't be as severe, but I went from twenty pills a day down to nothing.

What I tell other people in this situation is that going through withdrawal and treatment are probably the hardest things they ever have to do. Even if it is a tremendous shock to family and friends, most of them will eventually get over it and be supportive. I also try to impress upon them how important it is to not try to recover on your own at home. I tried it numerous times. Once I swallowed some pride and became humble enough to do whatever it took, I finally got the help that I needed.

Once in treatment, I quickly learned that everyone and everything else needs to be put on the back burner temporarily. I had to give up my kids for a month and a half to go to inpatient drug treatment. But what a blessing it has been in the long run. My life now is better than I ever dreamed it could be.

Perhaps the best way to explain what to expect in recovery is to relate exactly what happened to me. Every individual's experience will not be just like mine. After talking to many, many addicted people, however, I believe that there is a commonality in my story that binds us—all those who fight this fight—together.

My First Thirty Days
Day 1

My therapist had justification for admitting me to the hospital after seeing how depressed and high on pills I was both on that day and during several previous appointments. On that final day, I was so high on pills that my therapist wouldn't let me leave his office and asked me who he could call to take me directly to a treatment center for prescription medication abuse.

It's scary looking back on that time because I have very little memory of it. I remember only snatches of events, like stumbling down the hall in my therapist's office and sitting next to his desk, crying uncontrollably, unable to speak in complete sentences. I barely remember asking him to call my friend, Angela, to pick me up. While waiting for Angela, my doctor walked me out to the parking lot to make sure my car was securely locked. Yet, not only could I not remember where I parked my car, I couldn't remember the color, make or model. We walked around the office complex for about twenty minutes until I recognized it—parked nowhere near my therapist's office.

Six months earlier, Angela had expressed concern over my deepening depression and because I was showing signs of weight loss. She has since told me that she was not surprised by the phone call from my therapist. As she said, "I was afraid I would get this call one day." Since I remember little of that day, Angela has filled in the gaps for me. She told me when she arrived at my therapist's office, she was shocked at my appearance. Limp, pale, withdrawn and angry, I looked to her like a stranger. Gone was the independent and strong person she knew.

My doctor gave her my admitting papers for the treatment center before we left his office. On the drive there, Angela asked me what she should tell my husband, Michael. She also asked why I hadn't called him in the first place. I apparently told her I was afraid Michael would be angry and wouldn't understand. Angela promised to call him that night to let him know where I was.

On the way to the facility, I apparently kept trying to convince Angela that I needed to stop home for a few things—a change of clothes, a toothbrush and other essentials—but my therapist had told her to take me directly to the treatment center. He was afraid that if I got the chance, I would try to commit suicide or run away. He was right. I do remember feeling like that car ride was my last trip anywhere. I'm grateful Angela was there to help and kept me from sabotaging my chance at recovery.

Walking through the front doors of the treatment center, I felt butterflies in my stomach. Thoughts of running away to escape the unknown and the inevitable filled my head. I felt like everyone was looking at me, pointing fingers and judging me.

A pleasant receptionist greeted us and asked me to fill out admission forms. She also instructed me to give her my purse to be inspected for pills, alcohol and sharp objects, then it would be returned to me. A staff counselor came to escort me to her office to be interviewed and to assess my emotional and physical condition.

When I said good-bye to my friend, I felt alone and abandoned. I was in tears and scared. Thoughts of wanting to take more pills kept rushing through my head. Instead of listening to the counselor, I was trying to think of how I could manipulate this person into giving me the pills that were in my purse.

I felt frail and weak. I was weeping and trembling in fear, when I realized that my unsuspecting husband didn't even know yet where I was. Forgetting that Angela said she would call him later, I told the counselor my concern and she said they would notify him of my admission and why I was there.

I soon became too exhausted and lethargic from the dozen or more pills I had taken earlier in the day to move from the chair where I was sitting to a couch on which I wanted to lie down. The counselor attempted to continue her interview despite my overwrought state. She asked me when I last took a pill, what kind and how many. She asked if I felt suicidal and if I had memory loss. We discussed family history of depression. I was able to answer most of her questions until my speech became very slurred and I felt myself passing out on the couch. She immediately called in the facility admitting physician, who determined very quickly that I had overdosed. They transported me to the emergency room of the public hospital nearby.

After examination, the emergency room doctors realized that I was suicidal and that I had overdosed on several different types of pills as well as alcohol. Doctors quickly inserted a tube down my throat into my stomach. I gagged on the tubing and the charcoal used to induce vomiting. Emergency room doctors and nurses monitored my pulse and breathing for two to three hours while my counselor from the drug treatment facility stayed by my side. My wrists were shackled to the bed so I couldn't run away—which had definitely entered my mind.

Seven hours had passed since my last pill or drink of alcohol by the time I returned to the drug treatment facility from the hospital emergency room. Staff counselors escorted me to a specialized treatment area where patients begin their detoxification and where their conditions are monitored for any health emergencies that may arise.

The detox part of the facility had a very large carpeted sitting area with a television, a nurse's station, a meal room and bedrooms. Each bedroom had two beds and a bath and shower. I noticed the steel guard bars on the windows and doors with alarms that would sound if a patient tried to open any outside door in an escape attempt. I was completely exhausted from my ordeal at the hospital and more than ready to go to my own room and sleep.

Or so I thought. After the staff counselors escorted me to the specialized treatment facility, more strangers from the nurse's station came to me. They asked me to urinate into a cup to further check for drugs. This needed to be done with an open bathroom door—a precaution against suicide. Then they took my blood pressure, pulse rate and temperature. Then two female staff counselors escorted me to an examination room where they explained to me that they needed to do a search of my clothes for any drugs, alcohol or sharp objects that could put me or others in danger. They even took out my shoelaces. After getting dressed again, I was asked to lean forward while they ran fingers through my hair and checked in my mouth for the same reasons. While I felt as though I was a jailed criminal, these procedures, I learned, are all standard protocols in a treatment facility. Once they determined me safe, I was ready to retire to bed.

I thought I would be escorted to my room but, because my therapist left instructions that I was to be on suicide watch until further notice, I was not allowed to sleep in my room. Since I was required to have twenty-four-hours-a-day surveillance for seventy-two hours, I watched tearfully, too exhausted to argue at 3:00 A.M., as two staff counselors carried my mattress out of my bedroom to a well-lit hallway near the nurse's station. There, with loud noises, phones ringing, chatter and machines running, I didn't get much sleep.

Day 2

I somehow managed to get about two hours of sleep, only to be awakened by the 7:00 A.M. morning shift and early rising patients roaming the hallway past me. I could only use the bathroom if escorted by staff counselors, so I had to wait until it was convenient for them to take me. Everyone else was awakened shortly after 8:00 A.M. to start the day with breakfast, showers and dressing. Then followed group therapy, counseling and lectures on addiction. Patients too ill from withdrawal were excused from group therapy and cared for by nurses and staff. Medications were dispensed at the nurse's station by orders from a physician to help ease patients' physical pain, anxiety and depression.

On this day, my withdrawal symptoms began in the form of extreme nervousness and migraine. I felt chilled and clammy. I couldn't get comfortable in my own skin. I paced the floor and didn't want to converse with anyone. When the staff counselors noticed that I couldn't sit still and was crying uncontrollably, they asked my therapist to give me medication to calm my anxiety and help with my migraine. Having empathetic staff counselors with me in this time of crisis helped to ease the pain.

As I sat in a chair feeling worthless, my self-esteem in the gutter, a patient approached me who had been in the detoxification facility for a week. She said, "Hello, my name is Annie and I'm an addict." Annie put her arm around my shoulders as I cried. She told me I wasn't alone in this struggle and that I should focus only on this minute, hour or day. "We take one day at a time," she said. "We will love you until you can love yourself."

Annie had learned her wisdom through group counseling with other patients and individual therapy. Now that she was to be discharged soon, she needed to apply what she had learned to others. After Annie, other patients came to introduce themselves without judging my past or how I got there. I had already judged myself as being a bad person that didn't deserve anything good in my life. I had lost all respect for myself. I had jeopardized my marriage and lied and manipulated every one I knew in order to get pills. Still, the pills were on my mind, the only way I knew to "fix" the hell I was in.

Day 3

On day three, my withdrawal symptoms began to lessen and I silently sat in on a group therapy session.

Day 4

By day four, I was taken off suicide watch. I was relieved to have a room with a bed and bath that I could use without supervision.

Day 5

I went to a group therapy session, but I wasn't ready to share my feelings or trust anyone with my "secrets." It did me good to listen to others who did want to share stories of how they became addicted to their drug of choice. They told when, how and why they had felt drugs were needed. They told stories of emotional pain relating to their marriages, children and other family members. They described job-related pressures, depression, loss of self worth as well as physical and verbal abuse they had suffered. Tears rolled down my face as I thought how much I had in common with these strangers. It was as though we all lived the same life, same nightmare, same disappointments and fears. I was no different from these people, not any better, not any worse. I felt a new sense of belonging.

Day 6

Today was a good day. It can help boost your self-esteem so much when you become aware that your story is not so different from everybody else's.

Day 7

I woke up feeling irritable, jumpy and anxious. I was discovering how one day I could be up and the next day I could be down, just as the others said happened to them. This day the food didn't even look good. I looked in the mirror and didn't like the image looking back. I looked frail. I had no makeup and my hair needed styling. I was tired of wearing the few clothes I had brought with me.

Today I was to have a family counseling session with my husband, Michael, to discuss an "aftercare" plan before being discharged from the treatment facility.

This was not a good day physically for me, but emotionally I felt I was strong enough to continue my therapy at home as suggested by my therapist. Our family counseling session, however, left me feeling nervous, scared and unsure how Michael felt about having me back.

My husband asked what he could do to be supportive. I nervously watched him for any sign of distrust or anger toward me. I was very unsure of how he felt about having a wife who was a prescription medicine addict. Our communication skills had diminished over the years largely because I had been more interested in pills than in our relationship. I went home very nervous and unsure of our future together now that I was clean and sober.

Day 8

My first day home I felt as though I had entered into a dark cave. I felt claustrophobic in my own home. I felt like I was a stranger and I wasn't sure I belonged there. I saw through a kind of tunnel vision, as if I had a blind spot around all sides of my head and body. I could see only a few feet ahead of me. I could only concentrate for a few minutes at a time. I feared being alone and I was scared of doing something wrong now that I had been detoxed and was "alarmingly" sober.

I asked Michael to manage the medications my doctor had prescribed for anxiety and insomnia. My husband hid my medications from me and gave me my pills only as instructed on the bottles. I couldn't trust myself not to misuse them again.

Day 9

I was following the recommended treatment plan that had been written out for me on the discharge forms. I attended support groups every night as well as individual therapy. I still felt angry about allowing myself to get into this mess in the first place. I could not yet talk about my anger in therapy. But I was determined not to relapse.

Day 10

My husband began to attend Al-Anon, a support group associated with Alcoholics Anonymous where family members and loved ones of addicts share their stories, gain strength from each other and learn about the disease and themselves.

Days 11-15

With five more days behind me, I was now free of drug abuse for fifteen days! Fifteen days feels like months to someone newly in recovery. I had such feelings of pride and accomplishment. I had done what I was told to do, went to meetings, saw my therapist, stayed busy with activities and hadn't abused my prescriptions.

So why was I still depressed?

My withdrawal symptoms, like those of many other recovering addicts, continued after I returned home from the treatment facility. I would feel happy one minute, crying the next and snapping at my family and friends after that. I went from hyperactive to sluggish and back again. I felt angry that I wasn't feeling better faster. My emotional needs weren't being met and I didn't know what to do. The more physical and emotional pain I felt, the angrier I was for putting myself through this misery.

I didn't return to work after being discharged from the treatment facility. I was advised by my therapist to rest at home for a few weeks. I cleaned the house over and over, watched television and isolated myself from friends and activities. My husband and I were not getting along and we weren't communicating about anything "important." We didn't talk about my addiction or depression, and I didn't know where to begin to explain to him what had happened to me. I felt very alone and feelings of abandonment overwhelmed me. I couldn't understand what was happening to me.

Day 16

Today I was restless, confused and severely depressed with little hope of getting out of this doomed tunnel I felt trapped in. Michael was at work and my thoughts were muddled as to what was reality and what was not. I roamed the house looking for things to do to keep myself busy or amused. Then I found my thirty-eight-gauge revolver hidden in my closet.

I had taken lessons a long time ago and had enjoyed going to the shooting range, feeling the power of the gun as I aimed and shot at the target. I sat on the floor to open the case and took the pistol out. I looked at it for a long time, then stood up and walked down the hallway with the pistol in my hands, barely aware that it was there. The house was quiet and still. I walked to the kitchen and sat on the floor then leaned up against the wall. I remember thinking how pretty my pistol was as I held it in both hands.

Then without a thought in my mind, or reason, I pointed and placed the barrel of the pistol at my stomach. There was no fear, no thought of death, just a sense of calmness that I felt come over me. I never bothered to check first to see if the pistol was loaded. I discovered it wasn't loaded only after I pulled the trigger. I didn't realize what I had just done until I heard the gun chamber sound off the same as if it were loaded and ready to kill! Shaking and tearful, I sat quietly for what seemed a lifetime.

Still unaware of the full extent of my actions, I stood up, placed the pistol back into its case and put it back into my closet.

I didn't tell my husband about it when he came home from work. I pretended everything was fine.

Days 17-22

I attended my meetings for several days before divulging my secret about the pistol to my aftercare support group. My aftercare counselor notified my therapist of my episode with the gun. My therapist called me at home to check on me and do a phone assessment of my emotional stability. I was able to convince him that I was doing all right. I said I'd been feeling depressed and unable to communicate my fears to my husband. The therapist tried to convince me that perhaps I needed to be readmitted into the treatment facility for severe depression. I declined and told her I could work out my depression at home.

Day 23

I had gone twenty-three days without abusing or misusing prescription drugs! This is a monumental feat for anyone who has been addicted. Support group members acknowledge each other when they have been clean and sober for any length of time. The show of support from friends, family members, sponsors and church members can encourage the prescription addict to keep doing the next right thing: "to stay alive."

Twenty-three days of feeling full of life can make a person sharply aware of their surroundings. My hearing became clearer, flavors in foods were tastier, air smelled better, even water tasted cleaner. Things that most people take for granted became spectacular now!

A week had gone by without incident and I had put the gun scare out of my mind. I enjoyed going to my support meetings. I felt I fit in with the others who attended, even though I didn't fit in anywhere else.

Even so, I wasn't happy with myself and I had difficulty sharing my feelings with my group or anyone else, including Michael.

Days 24 through 30

Another long week passed without incident, without misusing or abusing any mood-altering chemical. Support groups have a "chip" (poker chip) system that acknowledges the number of days a person has been clean and sober. A person can receive a chip for thirty days, sixty days, ninety days, six months, nine months and twelve months. Those who are not prescription addicts or alcoholics don't always understand the significance, but we sure do! The day I received my thirty-day chip in my support group, I was overwhelmed with pride.

$$>>>7$$

FACING LIFE WITHOUT DRUGS:
*"Now that I'm sober,
I see that I don't have a life."*

The expression "get a life" seems made for the recovering addict. Once in recovery for a few weeks or months after abusing prescription drugs and no longer spending every waking moment trying to figure out new ways to get pills, recovering addicts are amazed how much spare time in a day they have. When you quit any habit, you immediately feel something is missing and boredom fills its place. Boredom is one of the strongest and most dangerous triggers for relapse. You must learn to recognize boredom before becoming prey to the cravings that inevitably accompany it.

It is understood that you are going to your therapist regularly and to your support groups often and you are in frequent contact with your sponsor. These interactions themselves take up time and at this stage that's good. Moreover, I cannot emphasize enough that therapy and support groups can be lifelines to peace and understanding without judgement or criticism. Your therapist will continually support and encourage your work toward recovery and your related achievements, no matter how small or large. He or she will listen when perhaps others won't. An experienced therapist does for you what you cannot do for yourself and what you will not be able to do for yourself for quite some time. You will face issues that you have avoided until now by misusing pills and you will learn the skills necessary to live a life that doesn't require prescription drug abuse to get you through the day.

At first, that's all you need to do—get through the day—but as soon as possible you need to start building a life. For many, that means starting from scratch. As for any building project, you need a plan, materials and some professional help to do the things you can't do yourself.

You may be thinking that you should just go back to work (if you worked before) or get a job if you haven't. Be cautious about this. Some, if not most, recovering addicts are not emotionally strong enough to go back to work during the first vulnerable weeks or months. Even if you need the money, try to make-do without going to work until you are truly ready, even if you have to beg or borrow money from family or take out a second mortgage on your home. If you go back to work too soon, you could be jeopardizing your recovery. If you can't stay sober under the stress of work, you will be back where you started and have to undergo treatment all over again. Please try to wait until you and your therapist together decide you can handle the challenges of going to work everyday.

Just as rebuilding your life does not mean going back to work, it does not mean making unnecessarily drastic changes in your world. No matter how tempting it may seem to reinvent yourself at this point, now is not the time to get married or divorced, change your job, buy or sell a house, move to the other coast or get pregnant. Research shows that even healthy people will get sick if the total life changes they experience within a year exceed a certain threshold. And an addict in early recovery is not a healthy person. Getting sober and giving up the habits of addiction are all the major changes you can take this year without risking other health problems.

Getting a Life

In making a plan for new possibilities and dreams, the first step is brainstorming your options. So sit down with some paper and pencil and do some exercises.

List activities that you once enjoyed before you became addicted. List the ones you did for fun—like ice skating, playing guitar, sketching or fishing— and the ones that were more like work—for example, studying a school subject, cleaning the house, pulling weeds or tinkering with your car. If you have trouble making a list, try to remember your likes and dislikes before you became addicted. To aid you in this task, ask yourself some questions: Are you good at making things with your hands? Do you like using words, reading or writing? Do you have musical talent? Do you like working with numbers and computers? Do you prefer talking with people throughout the day? If you've been addicted all your adult life, you may need to do some exploration to find your talents. Fortunately, there are books, classes and consultants to help you determine what you are good at and where your interests lie.

Approach these issues in different ways. Try writing out sentences like these below and then fill in the blanks.

I am a person who likes to...

I used to like to...

I don't want to do that now. I would rather...

Here's what stands in the way...

Here's how I could remove this obstacle...

Then list all the goals you remember having in the past. How many of these have you fulfilled? What are your goals now? Your number one goal, of course, is to remain sober. But what is your second goal? And your third?

Chances are you don't know the answers to some of these questions right now. You haven't been in recovery long enough. It's not too soon, however, to play with these ideas, see what gives your heart a little bounce, see what makes you sigh in despair. What turns you on, what turns you off? Make the effort to know yourself. And write your thoughts down in a journal. Writing helps clarify feelings, especially right now. You will also probably want to look back at your journal to remember your journey some day.

Don't wait for your whole life's plan to be formulated before you start living. Get busy now, keeping the idea of making a plan loosely in mind. Choose activities that soothe and strengthen your body, your mind and your spirit so that your whole self will heal.

Whereas at first you were just filling time with anything but drugs, now almost every activity should involve three key elements: **people, skills** and **purpose**. As you will see, one element leads quickly to another.

Meeting People

You need to be with people, because social interactions drown out the cravings in your mind as well as the doubts and negative thoughts. Spending time with others will also alleviate the fear and loneliness you feel as you continue on the bumpy road to recovery. The presence of friends and loved ones keeps you from looking around for drugs. Also, as you interact, you possibly are making up for years of hiding behind underdeveloped social skills. Your new interactions will help you learn to care about other people, share, be open, tell stories, listen, laugh and empathize.

You can choose activities that involve people by design (team sports, classes, workshops) or by invitation (walking with a friend, seeing a movie with your spouse, going to an art exhibit with your sibling.) You should do alone only those things you can be so engrossed in (reading, sewing or balancing the checkbook) that you don't get bored and let your mind wander. If you are bored, depressed or tempted, seek out people. Call a friend, call your sponsor, go to a group meeting, go somewhere where an activity is going on that you can join even if it's only taking your clothes to the Laundromat and washing them with the other coin-pushing folks. Ask a question of someone else who looks bored, start a conversation, offer to help someone fold their clothes while they are waiting. Interactions with people are your safeguard against boredom, the chief cause of relapse.

And don't forget that one special person in your life—your spouse or boy/girlfriend. Put "your song" on the stereo and ask, "May I have this dance?" Buy roses, cook a favorite dish or go to a restaurant you both enjoy. Buy a special nightgown; give a backrub. Remember the romance you had before your world revolved around pills and try to return to that time.

Developing Skills

An activity that builds a skill takes your mind off drugs as well as any other activity. At the same time, you build confidence. As you practice a new skill, you'll find that something you don't do very well (e.g. draw a picture, shoot a basket, start a conversation with a stranger) will become easier each time you do it. Simply having a skill gives you confidence. It is important to track your progress so you can see evidence of your increasing skill level, whether it means scoring higher, going farther while jogging or lowering your blood pressure. Keep a record of your progress in your journal.

A skill is a joy. A skill makes you proud. When you do something well, don't take it for granted; instead, say to yourself. "Wow, kid, you are not bad at all!" Besides the boost to your self-esteem, a new skill has practical value as well. You can use the skill around your house, on the job or share it with others.

One of the best ways to combine learning a new skill with social interaction is to take a class at a community center or continuing education program, join a sports team or lend a hand on a volunteer project. Thus you will not only learn new skills and gain new information, you also will benefit from spending time with **people**. More importantly, the new people you meet don't know your old untrustworthy self.

Gaining Purpose

At first, the purpose of your activities will be just to get you through the day while staying sober. As soon as possible, however, you should choose to do activities that include the three key elements: people, skill and purpose. Purpose includes short-term purpose and long-term purpose. Thinking about purpose, write your ideas down under the headings of the big areas of your life: **work, home, health, social life** and **spirituality.**

Work: Do you need new work goals? You may need less stress and therefore need to plan on changing jobs or on reducing stress in the job you have. Your activities could include or lead to courses necessary to change fields or jobs. For example, first, you might arrange for career guidance. This might be getting a book out of the library like Richard Bolles' *What Color is My Parachute?* or hiring a career consultant. It might mean taking an adult education class on choosing or changing careers. It might mean finding a program of education that leads to a new job skill or certification in a particular field or whatever you need to find a more satisfying job.

Home: Now that you are clean, you can begin to take pleasure in color, order, artistic arrangement. Do you want to make some changes in your environment to reflect your new upbeat take on life? Make a list of things you want to change around the house. For example, repair the ceiling and install a new light fixture, clean out and organize your closets and start a garden. For each project, write down the steps involved to accomplish your goal. Then break down the first step into little manageable steps you could do in one day. How about today! For fixing the ceiling, you could call your neighbor (Step 1) and ask who did their recent drywall work. You could go to the lighting store (Step 2) and look at fixtures. You could call the drywall contractor (Step 3) and ask him to come give an estimate. Or you could enroll in a class to improve your own dry wall installation skills. In the same way, you can break down the steps for reorganizing the closets or planting a garden. There are books in the library, consultants, specialists and classes to teach you to do just about anything you want to know how to do. Or you could team up with a friend with different skills than yours and do your project together.

Health: Getting clean was such a huge step toward better health that you may think you'll never need to do another thing. But building a life is about progress and improvement and reaching a higher level. It's time to revel in your new physical self.

Take an interest in your diet, read about healthy foods, go to a market that sells the freshest, most beautiful produce and learn some new, healthy ways to prepare them.

Exercise is paramount. Lying around for too long can bring on what we know as Stinkin' Thinkin', depression and relapse. Vigorous exercise actually changes your physical chemistry, giving you an adrenaline surge, lifting your spirits and lightening depression. Regular exercise reduces stress and tension. Aerobic exercise, like running, swimming, tennis and, of course, aerobics classes, lowers your blood pressure and heart rate. Other exercise, like yoga, dance and stretching, increases flexibility and mobility. Weight training enhances strength. With exercise you will feel more energetic and sleep better.

But how do you get yourself to do all—or any—of these things? How do you stay motivated?

Start an exercise program with other people. Join an aerobics class or hire a personal trainer. Buy a step-exercise video and invite someone to exercise with you in your home so you both stick with it. Join a rowing club; enroll in a martial arts class. Take up a sport you never tried, like ice-skating. Take up a sport you used to enjoy, like softball. There are "geriatric leagues" as well as youthful leagues in just about every sport. Buy a bike and explore the biking paths in your community.

All these activities cost some amount of money. If that's a problem, walk. (Ask for a gift of walking shoes for your birthday, Valentine's, anniversary or thirty days clean day.) Invite a friend to walk with you and get in a good visit while you walk. Walk to the library, walk to the bus stop, walk to work. Walk to the grocery store every day with a little pack on your back to bring your purchases home. Even if you have a perfectly good car, this daily routine—oh, so European—can provide the exercise and routine you need. If you live in a rural area or where the library and the store are too far away to walk to, instead go to the nearest mailbox to mail your bill payments or walk to your neighbor's house and bring something you baked. Walking just for exercise is extremely good for your health; walking with someone meets the goal of being with people; walking for a purpose meets another.

Remember that exercise is not solely comprised of rigorous activities like aerobics, weight lifting and hiking. Exercise can be going up the stairs instead of using an elevator or walking from room to room. Exercise can be vacuuming, sweeping, gardening or even dusting. Whatever forms of exercise you choose, get in the habit of doing something physical every day. Exercise will help keep you healthy, focused and toned.

Sometimes it's good to just pamper your body to relieve stress and make physical discomforts fade. Whether you indulge in a warm bath with scented candles or a treatment by a chiropractor, anything you do to keep yourself relaxed helps ward off stress-related discomfort and can sooth minor aches and pains so you don't feel the need to take a pill.

Some healthy alternative activities and treatments that heal your body while involving your mind and spirit include chiropractic, yoga, homeopathy, acupuncture, aromatherapy and massage.

1.   *Chiropractic* is the practice of healthcare management, primarily dealing with the recuperative powers of the body to heal itself without the use of surgery and/or drugs if at all possible. Chiropractors are the nation's third leading healthcare providers, exceeded only by medical doctors and dentists. The practice of chiropractic emphasizes the connection between structure and function. The chiropractic approach is based on the theory that adjustments to return the spine's alignment to its normal, healthy state will permit the nervous system to regain normal function, allowing the body to heal itself and eliminating pain and illness. Some chiropractors may supplement adjustment therapy with applications of heat, cold or electrical stimulation. They may also suggest lifestyle changes. Unlike doctors of osteopathy, chiropractors cannot prescribe medications.

2.   *Yoga* is the practice of mental and physical exercises to improve health. With yoga you use your mind and body to overcome obstacles both physical and mental. The word "Yoga" actually means, "disciplined," and it is through disciplined practice that many people have seen great results. Yoga encompasses specific behaviors, different breathing techniques, body postures and meditation. Age is not a factor when it comes to yoga. It's good for all people, regardless of their condition.

3.   *Homeopathy* is a two hundred-year-old practice of healing by the application of certain natural substances in minute amounts. The efficacy of tiny amounts of active ingredients is enhanced by a process of "shaking with impact" at each stage of dilution thus releasing the "dynamic energy" or healing information of the original substance. While the mechanism for healing cannot be demonstrated, healing effects have been documented by traditional medical research. Side effects, drug interactions, tolerance and addiction are unknown among users of homeopathic medicines. Homeopathic remedies are best when prescribed after a thorough interview of the patient by a homeopathic practitioner. A diploma or certificate from any homeopathic program by itself is not recognized as license to practice homeopathy in the United States. However, healthcare professionals—including medical doctors, osteopathic doctors, nurse practitioners, pharmacists, podiatrists and others—are permitted to use homeopathy within the scope of their state license to practice. Self-treatment with over-the-counter homeopathic remedies is safe, although perhaps not as effective as individualized treatment.

4. *Massage therapy* consists of rubbing, kneading, striking, tapping and stroking the skin and soft tissue for the promotion of health and the feeling of well-being. These techniques are great for the alleviation of headaches, tension, physical pain, injuries, chronic conditions and muscle soreness. Massage therapy stimulates blood flow and releases inflammatory or pain-producing substances, such as lactic acid, from the muscles. It helps reduce pain by relaxing muscles; by increasing lymphatic circulation, thereby reducing inflammation; and by promoting a sense of calm and relaxation. Techniques include acupressure, Swedish massage, deep-muscle massage therapy or rolfing and reflexology. However, check with your doctor before receiving any deep-muscle massage, because massage should not be performed on inflamed areas or on individuals with cancer or infectious conditions.

5. *Acupuncture* is an ancient Chinese procedure of relieving pain and treating an array of diseases through the use of needles. Specialists in acupuncture insert needles into specific points on the skin to relieve symptoms ranging from headaches to chronic pain to drug dependence. Researchers have demonstrated that the use of acupuncture produces an increase in the number of natural painkillers within the human brain and is useful in pain management and the maintenance of health.

6. *Aromatherapy* is a form of herbal healing. Scents and fragrances have been used for healing and mood change for thousands of years. Fragrant potpourri not only stimulates your senses, but lifts your mood, changing a bad mood into a good one in minutes. Simply by smelling or inhaling the active ingredients, you experience a physical change inside. Aroma consultants have recommended the following scents to alleviate depression and nervousness: melissa, narcissus, almond oil, sandalwood and lavender as relaxants, and chamomile, lemon oil, peppermint, spearmint, pine oil and rose as natural mood lifters.

When choosing an alternative therapy or practitioner, remember knowledge is power. Research credible healthcare information about any therapy you are interested in trying. Talk to people who have utilized the treatment method you choose to get recommendations for practitioners. Find out the practitioner's education, philosophy and years of experience. Inquire beforehand about charges for service, insurance coverage and policies on fees and payment. Call your insurance company and ask if your policy covers the alternative treatment.

Be responsible for your health and recovery. Evaluate your treatment and take part in deciding what should change and what should stay the same. Seek guidance from your healthcare provider, therapist, sponsor and peers for their viewpoints. Remember that not all treatments work for all people.

Social Life: Often, people don't think about how they got their friends. It may seem like the friends were made willy-nilly, as if chance threw them together. But each friendship starts with some kind of meeting. Write down all the friends you have and how you met each one of them. Now, **purpose** must be added to this activity. What is it you want to accomplish in your social life? Do you feel you need different friends or more friends? Perhaps the old ones have drifted away or they aren't supportive of your addiction recovery. Maybe they are old drinking or drug buddies who reinforce the bad habits you are trying to avoid.

If you decide you need to make new friends and develop your social life, you may worry that people you make an effort to meet aren't "real friends" because your relationship wasn't spontaneous. You may feel you need that spontaneous spark of connection to ignite a real friendship. However, after all the wasted time spent getting high on drugs, the recovering addict must put forth a serious, concerted effort to develop new, healthy friendships that aren't centered around drugs or alcohol.

Most important in your new circle of friends will be your support group. They will meet the requirement of understanding and accepting your addiction and recovery and they will take up a lot of your time. Pick and choose among this group the individuals you want to spend more time with outside of group meetings and whose company your spouse or partner might also enjoy. Once you feel you have made a connection, you can develop your friendship by inviting the person (or persons) to a movie, out to dinner or to join you for coffee before or after support group meetings.

As you move beyond needing every friend to be aware of your addiction, join unrelated interest groups. Take a variety of classes and when you find an area that really interests you, join an organization that promotes that interest, for example, a hiking club, a civic group such as Jaycees or Kiwanis, community theater or a pottery studio.

Friendships aren't the only damaged relationships in the lives of recovering addicts. Often, the most important relationships—those with spouses and family members—are badly in need of repair. First, you should tell your loved ones that you realize what your actions have done to them and that you are profoundly sorry. Then build your relationship just by being a healthy person when you are with them. It sounds simple, but it works. You don't have to do cartwheels or beg on your knees for forgiveness. Just be the person you wish you had been all along. Treat your spouse and family as well as you treat your new friends. Be honest and authentic with them. Invite them to join you in your new activities or for a pizza. Walk with them, go to a play with them, go to yard sales with them. Simply spend time with them. When they see the healthy, positive changes you have made in your life, trust will return and relationships will blossom.

If your purpose is still not clear, remember that you are still seeing your therapist while trying out these new ideas. You should talk to your therapist about how these new activities make you feel. Maybe the new activity brings about some new anxiety, maybe a person you chose to become friends with didn't want to be your friend or perhaps you find yourself skipping the new activity and sliding backwards emotionally. Tell your therapist. These are the kinds of things he or she is there to help with.

Spiritual Life: People who have undergone treatment for substance abuse often come through with a feeling of "renewal," a sense of well-being and inner strength. Some return to their original faith. Others question their original religion and find it doesn't seem to fit anymore. They may choose a new faith.

If you belong to an organized religion or at least did before your addiction, now's the time to strengthen it. Worship with your congregation. Read scripture or a daily devotional. Sing. Make a joyful noise. If you didn't have a spiritual life or don't now, be open to the spiritual possibilities around you. Spirituality need not come from organized religion only. It may come from a philosophy, point of view or activity different from anything you have considered or been exposed to before. Over a hundred different religions and beliefs in this world offer support, wisdom and guidance to those reaching out for inner peace.

In any case, religious or not, you should recognize that there is something more powerful than you are and that "something" is good. Any spiritual connection that comforts you and calls for a positive response on your part will lead you to grow spiritually. In twelve-step support group meetings, an expression often uttered is, "Let go and let God." The message behind the expression is that you must learn to let go of your problems and turn them over to God or whatever other higher power you believe in. Spirituality comes in many forms and can be very important to addiction recovery. If it gives you comfort, love, peace and strength, stay with it.

But if you are not there yet, don't despair. Readiness comes in its own time. Just be open to other beliefs, seek new experiences, learn from those around you and grow as a person.

Read Thomas Cahill's *The Gifts of the Jews* to learn about the historical beginnings of "the still, small voice." Read *Mere Christianity* by C. S. Lewis. Read *The Road Less Traveled,* the best seller by M. Scott Peck. Read the Twenty-third Psalm from the Bible out loud. Somewhere a line or a word or a story will touch you and set you on the path of spiritual growth.

All these activities of body, mind and spirit cross-connect, serving multiple purposes so that the whole healthy effect snowballs. To illustrate, here's one possible scenario: Your religious goal leads to singing in the choir and doing a helpful project for others. The one you choose is Habitat for Humanity, an organization that involves people like you building houses for the working poor under the direction of a skilled foreman. You are learning a new skill and getting hands-on experience. Your Habitat building skills and experience leads you to take up carpentry as a hobby and then to do carpentry for money. Next you leave the stress of your present job in a big office and become a carpenter working for yourself. Your new friends include the friends at church, the friends in Habitat, the friends in carpentry class and the people who hire you to do carpentry work.

Here's another possible chain of events: You decide you'd like a pet to ease loneliness, give purpose, etc. First your effort is very small. You read about pets and their care. You think you'd relate best to dogs. You read about breeds of dogs and their particular characteristics and temperaments. You choose one that you feel is best suited to your lifestyle. You read books on training and care of the breed you chose. After visiting the humane society and a few animal shelters to look at dogs available for adoption, you find you want to adopt. Training begins. As you walk your new dog around your neighborhood and the local park, you meet a lot of other dog owners. You're getting exercise and dogs attract people! You decide to go to a higher level of social engagement and sign up for an obedience class and then a course on agility training. Always you are making friends, practicing sobriety and learning skills that help you face life without drugs. The dog loves you in your good moments and your not so good times. You are forced to get out of bed every day, because you have a purpose: caring for your pet. Busy with new skills, new people and new purpose, you decide to become a dog groomer or trainer, or you and Fido visit the elderly in nursing homes for pet therapy. And it all started with reading a book on pets.

In these two examples, it is clear how one can go from filling time to getting exercise, learning skills, interacting with people and helping others. Though it takes time, you, too, can take the journey from nothingness to purpose. Every activity you engage in during your recovery has the potential of creating for you a social life, a growing skill and a new step on your purpose list. Life can be so joyful when you aren't thinking about escaping from it.

Maybe you're saying, *That all sounds very good, but I'm still lying in bed reading this book and I don't feel like getting up.* Yes, starting can be the hardest part. The first step needn't be a huge, overwhelming challenge. It can consist of simply picking up a sheet of paper and a pen or pencil. Now, with that small step out of the way, write down three goals. Then, for each goal, write down three activities that relate to that goal. Each activity should involve people, skill and the purpose of fulfilling your goal. For each activity, write down the first few little steps necessary to get started on that particular undertaking. Then get out of bed and do just one of those little steps. And then another...

You can use every activity you plan to do to make you feel more in control. Whether it's taking the winter clothes to the cleaners or just getting out of bed when you feel like lying there all day, if you plan to do it and follow through with your plan, your self-worth grows. When you have planned three things and accomplished those three things, you are three steps closer to your goal and three steps higher in self-esteem. Write down what you have done in your journal; mark the steps you have completed on your list with big red checks as you go. Reward yourself with simple pleasures like a hot shower, lighting a candle or calling a friend for a chat. You don't even have to wait for three completed steps to congratulate yourself. Do it after one step! It doesn't matter how small the step, it's the direction you go in and the regularity. You will get there. I know, because I have been where you are.

If and when you do go back to work, should you go back to the same job? Every situation is different. Are drugs available at work (e.g. in a hospital or doctor's office)? Were coworkers an enabling part of your drug-focused world? Is the stress of work such that you feel you have to have a pill, a drink or some other mood-altering substance in order to deal with it? If so, this job is not for you—not now.

Think hard about the stresses of your job that made you feel you needed a pill. What were the conditions at work? Were there personality clashes?

How much responsibility was put on you in a day? Too much? Too little? Were there long hours and poor management?

If you answered yes to most or all these conditions, then your risk of relapse could be high at that job and you should consider a change.

When you feel you are ready or you absolutely must work, look for a job, first of all, where drugs are not available. Also, seek a position with low stress. This may mean less responsibility or—if low responsibility represents boredom to you—more responsibility. Many drug users are looking for more risk and stimulation, higher activity levels and tighter deadlines, rather than less. If your most recent job was one you "stumbled into" without thought just because the job was available, this may be a good time for you to explore your job needs by reading books on choosing a career, taking a course on evaluating your work needs or seeking career counseling to determine just what kind of work environment you are best suited for.

Whether in a new job or an old one, now that you are focused and clear minded, you can perform your duties with greatly improved organizational abilities you never thought you'd have back. Your energy level will improve radically with this new and improved attitude on the job.

Nevertheless, every job comes with some stress. Think about possible changes you could make at work to reduce or avoid stress. This could include delegating duties to others or talking to your boss about working in a different department. Once you've made all the changes possible to reduce stress in your workplace, you must deal with whatever tension or pressure remains. You have to learn how to diffuse the stress and release your overwhelming emotions instead of letting them build up. Obviously, you can't use your stress-busting method of the past—taking drugs—so you must find an outlet for stressful anger or anxiety every day, like pounding a punching bag at the gym, doing aerobics, running, jogging, walking or dancing. Even yelling at the wall can release stress so you don't take it out on others or yourself. Take short (five minute) breaks at your desk for deep breathing exercises, stretching and meditation to refocus and relax your mind. Stress management is a learned technique that doesn't come naturally to everybody, which is why many people benefit from taking classes on the subject. Instructors teach students how to evaluate themselves and assess their feelings. They teach organizational and management skills that help individuals focus more clearly and make better decisions in stressful situations.

As for myself, even though I stayed in the healthcare field after my treatment, I chose not to return to the same clinic where I had worked before. That setting would have brought back too many memories of wrongdoing on my part, such as stealing sample medications, calling pharmacies for my own pills and the treadmill incident. Also, there I had to work under extremely stressful conditions with ten cardiologists and twelve employees. I decided not to return to a position that clearly could not be changed and no other position was available for me in that institution. Another reason for my decision was that I would always have felt guilty for letting them and myself down and for not giving them 100 percent. I couldn't look my old employers or colleagues in the face. I felt ashamed of myself and, perhaps, I still felt guilty. I have since gone back to apologize for my wrongdoing to a particular cardiologist with whom I worked for three years. I have found that letting go of the past is sometimes a good way to open your life to new possibilities and dreams.

After taking some of the basic steps outlined in this chapter, I decided to volunteer for the Red Cross. As a volunteer, I established relationships within the organization and proved myself as skilled, competent and reliable. When I was ready, I took a new job as a health educator for the Red Cross, where I continue to work today.

My husband and I, through a combination of joint counseling, talking and listening to each other and trying hard to be better individuals, have built a more solid, stronger marriage then we ever imagined possible.

In my spare time, I pursue my passion, which is to help other prescription drug addicts recover and to educate people about prescription and over-the-counter drug abuse. When I could not find a support group specifically for prescription drug addicts, I started one called Prescription Anonymous in my hometown. I have gone to other states to help form chapters and will continue this work until there are groups available all over the country. In addition to sponsoring two recovering addicts, I have been lobbying my state legislature to pass a new "Bill of Rights" requiring selected drugs to carry warning labels about their addictive natures. I would like the labels to say: "If you are an individual recovering from chemical or substance abuse, supervision should be used while taking this medication."

These interests and activities have filled my life with positive stimulation and a sense of peace, so I no longer need uppers, downers or chemical mood alteration of any kind. I am aware that I will always be an addict and can always relapse if I make a mistake. But the fullness of my life makes me feel that I have come a long way and can achieve success in my battle. Write to me through Prescription Anonymous, Inc. and tell me how you have achieved success, too.

RELAPSE:

*"I'm in recovery,
but I'm still an addict."*

Relapse is a constant fear for the recovering addict. I believe it is a healthy fear, because that sense of dread keeps you safe. You never want to forget the chaos and pain this disease has brought you. Remember, however, that relapse can become a learning experience that makes you stronger. If you are willing to try sobriety again, a relapse can bring you closer to real life-long recovery.

My relapse occurred after I had been released from the treatment facility and detoxed from my various drugs. After a while, I realized I had suffered the pain of withdrawal without winning back happiness. This realization made me quit caring about recovery. I began to talk myself out of my new state of sobriety. Then I talked myself out of life altogether. This was before I was diagnosed or realized I was suffering from depression as well as addiction and I needed to be treated for both. When a half-hearted attempt to kill myself failed, I took some pills I had squirreled away before my "recovery" and then, only when I was in relapse, did I call my therapist.

A relapse is a slip out of sobriety. The prescription addict's definition is stringent: the use of any mood or mind-altering substance or medication, over-the-counter or prescribed, not exactly according to a fully informed physician's directions. It's a zero tolerance definition. There is no judgment factor such as "too much" or "too often," or even "unknowingly." Note, however, that some people, even some addiction support groups, say that if you're on any kind of pill, you have relapsed. This is not true. Just as diabetics need their insulin, people with elevated blood pressure need medicine to control it and people with heart problems need their stabilizing medication, so prescription addicts with a dual diagnosis often need prescribed drugs to combat depression or anxiety, combined with behavioral therapy. If left untreated, such mental illnesses greatly inhibit the addict's recovery. The point is that any medication taken must be prescribed by a competent physician to whom you have told the truth. Medication taken under any other circumstance constitutes relapse.

Why would a person who has suffered the discomfort of withdrawal ever relapse? There are many reasons, but basic among them is the lack of sufficient motivation going into treatment and inexperience in recovery.

Lack of motivation may be the obstructive factor in long-term recovery because the person was forced into treatment and did not come of his own volition. He simply wasn't ready. While many who are forced or persuaded by a loving intervention to enter a treatment center do "come around" and commit themselves to recovery, many others are just going through the motions to satisfy someone else.

Marilyn, one relapsed addict, speaks for those like her: "In treatment we were always doing what was expected of us to make everything 'alright' again. We did what we thought others wanted us to do—our spouses, family, children or employers. We were in recovery for everyone but ourselves. When we tried it again *just for us*, that was the turning point."

Some recovering addicts relapse, even though they are motivated, because they are motivated to do many things. Unfortunately, recovery takes so much of your energy and attention that concentrating on other things in your life causes you to neglect recovery. Often, addicts don't realize they can't successfully go through a recovery program and do all the other things they are motivated to accomplish.

"When you put everything before recovery, you will lose to this disease," says Marie, a member of Prescription Anonymous. "I put everyone else first—my husband, kids, in-laws, business—thinking that if I made them happy, I would be doing the right thing. I knew I had turned the corner when I put recovery as my first priority."

Some enter into treatment knowing they have a stash of pills hidden at home "just in case." This kind of doubt gnaws at the recovering addict's commitment. One woman who felt she couldn't go into a treatment center had worked it out with her husband that he would give her the pills less and less frequently until she was taking no more. "I really want this to be the end of it for good," she said, explaining the procedure, but adding, "I still have three refills left that I can always get from the pharmacy if it doesn't work out." She is setting herself up for relapse by even thinking about those refills. Truly sincere commitment means flushing your remaining pills down the toilet or telling a responsible person where all your reserves are hidden so they can dispose of them before you come home. Then the drugs aren't even there to see or think about.

Even if an addict was motivated during treatment and felt positive about his future free of drug addiction, he may suffer from overconfidence coming out, thinking, "I'm recovered." This individual will not be prepared for the difficulties that lie ahead, because he is inexperienced. Inexperience is the cause of poor judgement in any area of life, so why assume it will be different for addiction recovery? It takes learning, then trying, making mistakes and correcting them before any new process is mastered.

Overconfidence may also indicate a newly recovered addict's deeper layer of denial. In this case, the individual thinks she's learned all she needs to know to stay clean and sober, so she is careless in her behavior. She may not observe all the necessary precautions. The likelihood of relapse for this person is great.

Addiction specialist John Wallace, M.D. says, "Recovering individuals must gradually change their patterns of thinking. Just as denial has enabled addicts to persist in self-destructive, pill-taking behavior counter to their values, its continued use after they stop their abuse can leave them vulnerable to relapse. Sometimes, after a prescription addict has been detoxed and is beginning to feel better physically, he mistakes a craving for pills for a reasoned assessment that he can now take charge and medicate himself as needed. With this deception, he fools even himself."[1]

One forty-four-year-old relapsed addict, Scott, explains how he deceived himself into believing he could take pills and still be in control.

I stayed clean for nearly two years. Then, just when I thought I had it licked and had all the answers, I relapsed. I thought I had been cured! I thought I could use just a 'little' and not let it get out of hand. Well, my thinking got me right back into the living hell of drug addiction.

I am working now at getting back on the road to recovery. I have faith that, if I stick with it, I can live a life free from the insanity of drug addiction. I have learned a valuable lesson: recovery from drug addiction is not easy. It requires honest effort. The rewards, though, are priceless!

Scott's reason for relapse is now clear to him. He won't make that mistake again. His motivation is great, probably greater now, after relapse, than the first time around. This is why I believe that relapse is not necessarily failure. It is a distinct stage of change rather than failure to change. It is a signal that more change is necessary. You relapse until you get it right. If relapse is approached appropriately, it results in a renewed and refined effort at change. Part of the process is to obtain more knowledge about addictive behavior patterns and to learn the new behavior patterns necessary for a healthy, sober life.

This isn't just a matter of opinion. Studies indicate that most people treated for any type of substance dependency relapse at least once and a significant number experience two or more relapses. Between one-half and two-thirds of addicts in treatment will relapse within one year. According to Terence Gorski, president of The Cenaps Corporation, a prevention training organization, "One-third of all patients are recovery-prone and maintain total abstinence. Another third are transitionally relapse-prone and have series of short-term and low-consequence relapse episodes prior to finding long-term abstinence. The final third are chronically relapse-prone patients who can't find long-term sobriety no matter what they do."[2] The belief that relapse is an indication of weakness or failure belies the fact that, for many people, successful recovery often involves a series of relapse episodes.

Treatment after relapse feels different from the original treatment. The first time an addict enters treatment, he usually doesn't have any real idea of what will happen, including how withdrawal will feel. All he knows is that he wants to feel better and end his dependence on drugs. He is fearful but hopeful about the future. First time recovery treatment is a "learn as you go" process.

On the other hand, treatment for relapse feels worse than the first time in several ways. Now the addict knows what's going to happen to her. She dreads the aches, shakes and nausea. Moreover this feels even more like failure, because she has not only let herself down, but she has let the loved ones down who supported her through this ordeal once, twice or six times before, only to have to do it all over again. The unhappiness over her failure increases the risk of depression for the addict receiving a repeat treatment. She may have thought when she went into treatment the first time that all she needed to do was detox, go to a few meetings, say the right things and that's all there was to it. It's a rude awakening when she finds she has relapsed.

Treatment after relapse is where the real work begins. The good news is that the second treatment can make the addict stronger, more focused and more determined to make sobriety the first priority. Relapsed members of support groups say that when they returned to treatment they learned something new and valuable about themselves and the process of staying in recovery. They listened harder and retained what they heard. As if watching a movie for the second time, they picked up new information they had missed or forgotten.

This is not to say that you should try to relapse! Relapse is not fun. But if you do relapse, try to consider it something you evidently needed to do, forgive yourself and learn from the experience. Whatever you do, don't assume relapse means you've failed. The odds of maintaining life-long sobriety are still in your favor. Keep fighting!

Whether you realize it or not, recovering addicts set themselves up for relapse days or weeks before it actually happens. A series of changes in behavior and thinking in recovering addicts allows relapse to happen. In response to a gradual progression of "warning signals" that herald emotional pain, addicts talk themselves into the inevitability of abusing prescription or over-the-counter drugs again. As a result, they believe they are unable to function without pills or some other mood-altering substance. By self-medicating, they return to what they know will diminish or mask their emotional or physical pain. Here are some of the self-defeating thoughts that, given a few hours or days to work on the recovering addict, will often result in relapse:

> *I don't deserve to be happy.*

As the recovery process begins to make you feel better about yourself, you may start feeling a little guilty about being happy. After living in a world of self-destructive behavior then changing for the better, you will feel different, both physically and mentally. Many addicts have difficulty dealing with change and, as a result, they question why they should be happy.

To answer this self-defeating question, tell yourself that you deserve to be happy because you faced your addiction and are working hard to be a better person. Then, do something good, productive and worthwhile, so you can show yourself in a tangible way why you are deserving. This exercise is especially effective and meaningful if you do something for someone other than yourself, so that the other person's gratitude and appreciation will act as external validations of your worth.

> *I can't go another day; it's just too hard.*

There will be times when you feel like you can't stand another day of being miserable. When you feel like this, get out of the house. Visit a friend, do some gardening, see a movie, etc. The worst thing you can do is be alone.

No matter what the cause of your unhappiness, share it with others. Call your sponsor or a close friend. Allow them to help you shoulder the burden of your pain and sadness—at least temporarily. Most importantly, banish the words, "I can't," from your vocabulary. Every time these words enter your consciousness, stop what you're doing and tell yourself, "Actually, I *can* do it and I know I can because I have been drug-free for seventeen (or however many) days already and I am proud of it."

> *I feel like I'm in a dark tunnel of depression. I hate it.*

Depression can be a very difficult emotional problem to deal with, whether a person is a recovering addict or not. Depression makes you feel utterly alone, as if the world has forsaken you to live in a dark tunnel, and makes you believe there is no relief in sight for your sadness and pain. Take it one minute at a time; try not to focus too far in the future because it is often too overwhelming to handle. Look on your calendar and find your next appointment with your therapist. Say, "Only three days until I see her. I can make it until then." If there is no such appointment on your calendar, make one now. In fact, it's good to always have an appointment out there in the future. You can always cancel it (giving sufficient notice as a courtesy) if you are feeling good. The dark tunnel does eventually open wide and disappear, letting light in and allowing your mind to become clearer and more focused. When good feelings begin to overtake the bad, you will feel more confident with yourself and proud of every hurdle you get through. The light at the end of the tunnel is closer than you think.

Common Triggers

Besides relapse-inviting, negative thoughts, the National Institute on Drug Abuse states, "Other factors can be entangled in relapse, including difficult life experience, lack of a support system and an inability to handle stress. The inability to learn skills to manage stress is a major relapse trigger in recovering individuals."[3]

We can increase our chances of not relapsing by recognizing the dangerous feelings we call triggers and knowing actions we can take to cope with them. Triggers will be different for everyone depending on their backgrounds, childhoods, self-images, how and why they started taking drugs, etc. To get an idea of the different triggers that cause relapse in real people, I asked some recovering prescription addicts what thoughts and behaviors preceded their relapses and came up with the following list of the most common triggers.

Cravings

It was the cravings that got me. I couldn't get them out of my head. Once I was back home from treatment, I didn't have anyone there who understood how I felt.

Sometimes relapse is a simple response to intense cravings. Emotional memories are our deepest, most powerful recollections; they can often be evoked by some sensory cue like a taste or a smell and they seem to shortcut the process of rational thought. Post-traumatic stress disorder (PTSD) leads to the most dramatic manifestations of emotional memory. For people with this syndrome, even small cues can bring the entire traumatic episode flooding back to awareness with all its original emotional intensity intact. Similarly, long after all symptoms of withdrawal from drugs have faded, "the body remembers," says Dr. Anna Childress of University of Pennsylvania Treatment Research Center.[4] The individual "desires" to recapture the mind-altering experience and to relive it again and again and again. Thus, at the same time drugs commandeer the brain's wiring, they lay the bedrock for powerful emotional memories that stimulate cravings and therefore tempt the addict to relapse.

Cravings can be more frequent and intense in the first several weeks or months of recovery. Cravings can leap into your head at any moment without warning. The best way to protect your sobriety from cravings is to track them. Keep a log of when and how often the cravings come. Write in your journal where you were and what you were doing when each craving hit. For example, what sights, sounds, smells and tastes were you experiencing when the craving hit? What mood were you in when your craving began? Then, write down what you did to alleviate the craving or get your mind off it. How did you avoid giving in to the craving each time? Once you have a record, you can study it and learn to recognize the dangerous moods and sensory experiences that trigger cravings and the most effective ways you've been able to ward them off. You can then start to develop a system to intervene when the craving strikes and do what works to help you avoid giving in, whether it means calling a friend or sponsor, going to a support meeting or just getting out of the house to take a walk.

Boredom

I had too much time on my hands while I was at home. I was left alone all day, feeling bored and lonely. I had all this free time and nothing to do to replace my thoughts of abusing again.

Stay busy with hobbies, meetings and exercise. Seek out people with whom you feel safe, enjoy socializing with and who make you feel like re-engaging life again. Contact those friends who have a positive influence on you or call friends from your support group.

Depression

I can't seem to snap myself out of this dark tunnel I feel I'm in. I cry and isolate myself to the point that I have difficulty motivating myself to do anything.

Some people know the reasons for their depression. In the past, they may have used pills to mask feelings they didn't want to think about or deal with. While in recovery, they had to face up to those negative emotional problems without the aid of a pill. That can be incredibly difficult and painful for anyone to handle, even those who aren't prescription addicts. It is important to talk about these feelings and problems openly and honestly with people who care about you. Ask your therapist to help you solve the underlying problem.

Sometimes, however, people don't know why they are depressed, they just know they are. They know of no specific problem that needs solving and thus don't know what to do to feel better. When this vague depression strikes, one of the best methods of dealing with it on your own is to use relaxation skills learned through activities like yoga or engage in some activity that provides peace and satisfaction. In addition, safe, appropriate doses of medication, prescribed and supervised by a physician, may be necessary. Talk to your psychiatrist, therapist, sponsor or support group.

Anger

I felt angry all the time. I was angry with my wife, kids, neighbors, co-workers and even the family pets, everyone but myself. I wanted to blame others for my addiction.

Anger kept bottled up inside is a relapse waiting to happen. Anger can not only cause relapse, but it can destroy you, your marriage, your family and other relationships. Nothing positive can come from misdirected anger. Work through it with your therapist, support group, sponsor, spiritual advisor or a good friend you respect. When an attack of anger strikes, go for a hard work-out at the gym or a brisk walk, clean the house or mow the lawn. Burn off some anger by putting it to good use rather than by hurting others or yourself.

Bad habits

I went back to the same friends I had before. They were still using drugs. When I wasn't with them, I found myself going through other friends' medicine cabinets and purses to steal their medications. It was so easy for me to do.

Socializing with the same crowd of people who also misuse pills or alcohol can only make things worse for you and you will probably relapse because of it. Make a list of these people and put them off-limits! Bad habits also include lying and stealing. To hide your drug addiction in the past, you probably became very adept at lying to your spouse, boss, co-workers, friends, physician, dentist and pharmacist. Now, every time you go to a healthcare provider, before you are even tempted to lie, you must tell them up front that you're a prescription addict. This will help them see through you if you slip into the old lying habit and they will make every effort not to give you any mind-altering medications. Ask your very good friends and understanding relatives not to leave their purses or prescriptions around unattended or within easy reach for you.

Low self-esteem

I had a difficult time restoring my self-esteem and self-worth and I didn't get any help or support from my family. I felt so ashamed of what I had done to myself and others.

When you have very low self-esteem, it is difficult to be motivated to improve. And, though self-worth comes from within, it certainly doesn't help to be surrounded by negative, critical people. It is important to make an effort to spend time with positive, supportive, happy people. Perhaps, if you have difficulty finding positive people in your current everyday life, you can reestablish a relationship with a friend from years past who was always upbeat and positive. Healthy relationships can help to restore your self-worth and motivate you. Another simple activity you can do is write down a list of all your good qualities and all the things you have done that you're proud of. Read this list when you are feeling really down about yourself. Self-esteem can get a boost from affirmations and acknowledgment of your good points. But the straightest, strongest route to self-esteem is to earn it: Do a task well, be kind to others, stay sober. It won't take long for people to notice your efforts and let you know how much they appreciate you. These are the reinforcements you need to increase your self-worth. Win them by good behavior.

Criticism

I never get positive feedback from my spouse or family. I always hear "You'll never amount to much in life" or "Why can't you be more like your brother? He's successful." I got high on pills so I wouldn't have to think about their comments. It was easier to not feel anything.

Criticism is tough for anyone to take. It's especially easy for prescription addicts to believe the negative things said about themselves and not hear or believe the positives ones. It is as if they don't feel they're worthy of any positive things said about them. Instead of feeling badly and agreeing with people when they say negative things about you, consider how unhappy those people must feel being burdened with all those negative thoughts. Think of criticism as one of *their* bad habits, not a reflection of who you are. Concentrate on getting rid of your own bad habits and building a healthy lifestyle. The healthier you become, the happier and more worthy you will feel.

Family disapproval

My family members are my biggest triggers. They can depress me, anger me, frustrate me, bore me and accuse me of God knows what, all within seconds after I walk into a room. Before, I'd take a pill to protect myself against them. They still make me think about taking a pill.

Distance yourself from anyone who cannot be positive and supportive—even if it's a family member. You are not punishing them; you are just protecting yourself. Once you are well into your recovery and you feel that you can help negative people to be more understanding, then approach with caution. Don't expect miracles, but in time they may listen and be supportive as they see the changes in you. If they don't ever approve of you or agree with you about your changed behavior, that is their choice and right. While you're around them (if you choose to be), change the subject from your illness to the wonderful things happening in your life. The more energized and happy they see you are, the more they will let go of their disapproval and admire the person you have become.

Facing People

People at work kept looking at me like I was going to lose my cool or sell them drugs. I couldn't stand being treated as if I was a criminal. My best just didn't seem good enough.

Facing people who knew you before recovery can be difficult. You feel like you're walking on eggshells, not knowing how to act or talk around people, fearing their judgement and criticism. Be patient with people. They have seen your bad behavior before and they are not sure how your new behavior is going to work out. Can you blame them? Just keep doing the right things by staying away from pills, going to meetings and showing that you are truly worthy of being trusted. Remember, they may feel as though they're walking on eggshells, too, because they don't want to say or do anything that might upset you. Communication is the key. Keep everything out in the open and help each other to understand what's going on.

Not going to meetings, therapy or utilizing sponsor
I got tired of going to meetings and counseling and having to meet with my sponsor all the time. I felt like that was all I had in my life: everyone else telling me what I should do, where I should go and when I should do it.

Stopping support group attendance, therapy sessions and frequent contact with your sponsor will undoubtedly push you to relapse. When you are new in recovery, you need close supervision, support and structure, whether you like it or not. You need to learn how to change bad habits into good habits. Recovery is hard work, because changing old behaviors doesn't come easy. You need feedback, encouragement and guidance. "Working a program" alone—without any help whatsoever—didn't work for me and likely won't work for you, but meetings, sponsors, good friends and therapy do help if you let them.

I cannot emphasize this enough: You must stick with therapy, your support group and your sponsor. The people telling you what to do have at one time been right where you are now. They know what you're going through better than anyone else. And they know what lies ahead for you. They have only your best interests in mind. You will come to know how important they are and learn to enjoy being around them. People in meetings not only learn about their disease and get to share their concerns with each other, they also find new friendships. These people become your "partners in recovery" and your friends. You will always need a support system to help with the bad days and to share the good days and that's what these people will become.

Guilt and shame
I was consumed with guilt and shame over what I had done to my family. I hurt my wife so much by lying that I couldn't face her. Also, I was in

a car accident while under the influence of over-the-counter medicines and injured two people. I can't forgive myself for that.

The predators of guilt and shame have been living inside you for months, maybe years, and they will gnaw at you to the point of destruction if you let them. Talking about your guilt and shame in meetings and attending family counseling can help you work through these feelings until you find the answers you need to put the past in the past and move on to a better future. Don't let guilt and shame destroy you as many have. Learn to ask for help and open up to others who want to see you succeed. Beware: guilt and shame don't go away over night; you must be patient with yourself and others while you work through this. As you do, be gentle and respectful to those you feel you have hurt. Making amends is a powerful step in the recovery process and is a part of many twelve-step programs. You'll feel relieved that you have confronted your mistakes. You can't change the past; you can only change the present. Guilt and shame will diminish as you begin doing more things of which you can be proud.

Physical pain

My physical pain was so intense that I felt justified taking extra pills. I followed the instructions on my prescription bottles, but I also went to the pharmacy and bought sleeping aids so I could get through each night without pain. That caused my relapse.

When confronted with pain, prescription addicts often associate their discomfort with an immediate urge to take a pill. They think, "I can't stand this feeling any longer. I have to have a pill." In fact, since pain in the past has led to the sweet relief of medication, addicts are often conditioned to feel discomfort or pain in order to justify taking the medication. This is a connection addicts need to unlearn. When that first sensation of discomfort hits, you need to engage in a distracting activity to disrupt the unhealthy link between pain and your desire to pop a pill.

That said, I believe no one, not even a recovering addict, should have to suffer intense physical pain. You can have medication for pain—the right medication, prescribed by the right people and taken as directed. Your therapist, addictionologist and pharmacist understand addictive medicines. They should be the people who tell you what medication to take and how much to take so that the risk of relapse will be low. Listen to their instructions and do what they tell you without deviating. Until you have proven you can trust yourself, ask your spouse or some responsible person to keep your prescribed medications locked up and to administer them to you only according to the doctor's instructions. **Never** self-medicate without supervision and that includes over-the-counter medicines! When you self-medicate, you are in relapse.

Availability

Going to any healthcare provider, dentist or pharmacy was like going to a candy store and pressing my nose against the glass. Everyone has a medicine cabinet in their house just asking to be opened. And every medicine cabinet has got something that looks good to me.

Availability of drugs is a real problem, especially since all your friends and even the people you live with probably have dozens of medications they legitimately need or that are left over from a previous illness. Here's the solution: Ask your spouse, partner or whomever you live with to clean out the medicine cabinet now or before you come home from treatment. This is not a do-it-yourself project for you. Ask someone to comb the house for pills you may have stashed away. Tell this person to check behind the window blinds, in the toilet tank, in your clothes pockets, purses, in jars in the kitchen and in other places only you know about. You don't want to stumble upon an old cache of pills when you are newly sober.

Ask others in your household to put their own medicines in a locked container and to keep the key with them. That's an inconvenience for them, but nothing compared to the inconvenience of living with an addict in relapse.

And I repeat, tell your doctors and other healthcare workers that you are an addict or that you have an addictive personality. It's essential for you to communicate with all healthcare professionals about your addiction and to feel confident these professionals know how to prescribe non-addictive medications. Ask your doctor for the diagnosis, not just the symptoms. Ask that you be involved in the decisions for any necessary prescriptions. We live in a world where it has become automatic to be seen by a healthcare provider and handed a prescription without even discussing the addictive components of the medication or whether your symptom is one that is "short lived" and can be managed without drugs. Doctors have become accustomed to writing out prescriptions for tolerable symptoms without patients even asking for them. Make the choice be yours. Can you treat your symptom without running the risk of relapse? Is the prescription offered written for a passing symptom or for the root cause of a significant disease? Remember, don't let your addiction "trick" you into unnecessarily putting a pill into your mouth.

Over-the-counter Drugs and Relapse

Many people never think that over-the-counter medicines are as addictive as prescription medications. Yet over-the-counter stimulants such as diet pills, caffeine tablets, nose sprays, sedatives that contain alcohol, sleeping aids and cold remedies all can be potentially dangerous. Nan Davis, R.Ph., M.S., pharmacist and founder of Pharmacy Counseling Services, says, "It is difficult to live drug free in a society flooded with quick-fix drug advertising. Sometimes, it seems almost un-American to endure aches and pains without doing something about them. Breaking the pattern of impulsive drug use may necessitate the removal of all medications from the home. Unfortunately, long-standing, compulsive drug seeking and supply procurement behaviors make it difficult to clear the home of drugs. Common excuses for keeping drugs include: 'I might need it someday,' 'It's for somebody else,' and 'But it's not addicting.'"[5]

Davis explains that pharmacists, like physicians and dentists, need to be aware of the potential dangers of prescription medication and over-the-counter drugs for their patients in recovery. Any mood or mind-changing drug taken to relieve anxiety or other discomforting symptom in a prescription addict or alcoholic results in relapse an unacceptable percentage of the time. Pharmacists understand and can explain the mechanism of non-drug and drug-minimum alternatives, though some may need education updates on how their drug knowledge applies to addiction and recovery. As respected professionals, pharmacists and dentists, as well as physicians, have a special responsibility to assist recovering alcoholics and addicts to use medication appropriately. For example, if a pharmacist is asked "Can you help me find medicine without alcohol that will treat my cold?" he should take time to explain the potential psychoactive side effects in both liquid and solid dosage forms of any medicine he recommends. Rather than resorting to a systemic agent with potentially undesirable side effects for a recovering addict, the pharmacist could recommend a vaporizer and explain the effects of increased fluid intake and even inhaling the vapors of hot chicken soup.

The risk of adverse drug effects is generally acceptable only if the disease being treated is in itself very serious. Use of a potentially addictive drug for a trivial illness, however, is unacceptable, considering the high risk of relapse.

This is not to suggest that people in recovery should never medically use drugs again. Many have been safely used with proper precautions. The trick is to use the least addictive form of a necessary medication that will be effective and to follow your doctor's or pharmacist's instructions carefully.

The most addictive nonprescribed and prescribed medications fall into three categories: stimulants, narcotics and sedatives. Stimulants cause the central system to speed up and they also suppress hunger. Narcotics can cause a momentary rush or pleasurable feeling as well as pain relief. Sedatives slow the body down, cause drowsiness and temporarily relieve anxiety, worry, depression and nervousness. Stimulants, narcotics and sedatives are all available in small amounts in certain over-the-counter medicines.

As an addict, you should never purchase an over-the-counter medication on your own. Other people may buy over-the-counter drugs without harm, but not you. A mouthwash you might consider harmless will probably contain alcohol, a mood-altering drug you may not be able to have even in small doses. Diet pills often contain stimulants to make the dieter burn off extra calories; these often lead to the use of stronger stimulants like amphetamines. A cold or sinus medication may contain pseudoephedrin, an effective decongestant that also acts as a stimulant. Banned for Olympic athletes, pseudoephedrin should also be banned for the recovering addict.

If your healthcare provider or therapist has diagnosed a symptom that requires an over-the-counter medicine and they have <u>prescribed this medication to you</u>, then, and only then, should you purchase it. Realize that for prescription addicts there can be no absolutely safe list of medicines. Listed below, however, are a few non-addictive medicines, suggested by pharmacists as reasonably safe for you and the symptoms or ailments these medicines treat.

HEADACHE	Aspirin, Extra Strength Tylenol, Bufferin, Advil, Aleve
STOMACH ACID, NAUSEA	Pepto-Bismol, Emetrol, Nausetrol, Emecheck
NASAL CONGESTION	Ocean, Humist, Ayr, Saline, Nasal, Salinex
SORE THROAT	Vicks Chloraseptic, Sucrets lozenges, Vicks cough drops
MOUTHWASH	Cepastat
COUGH/COLD	Naldecon Senior EX, Robitussin (not DM), Breonesin Capsule
INSOMNIA/SLEEP AIDS	Chamomile tea, Sleepy-time tea, warm milk

I have devoted pages to the use of over-the-counter medication by the prescription addict because, while a great many relapses are triggered by such factors as boredom and anger, prescription addiction still is a disease of drug abuse. Having clear rules about what substances you can have and what to stay away from is basic to recovery. Using medications not prescribed for you or misusing any similar substance is relapse.

When will you know you are out of the woods and you will not be facing relapse again? One answer is NEVER.

As Teresa explains after several years of recovery, "I still go to support groups, not only for chronic pain but also for addiction, because I am still petrified that one day I may take a Percocet and I'll be back where I was years ago. The support groups help me remember where I was and where I want to be."

Another answer is SOME DAY.

Remember Carol, who detoxed and recovered under a doctor's supervision without her husband ever knowing she was addicted? Here, Carol reveals how she knew she'd "made it:"

My husband had dental surgery recently and will have to have it again in a few weeks. The dental surgeon gave him a prescription for the same painkiller I had been addicted to. I had to go to the same drugstore where I had gotten many of my refills to have his prescription filled. Then I had to carry the pills home, bring them to my husband with a glass of water and watch him swallow them. He has no idea these pills might be a temptation for me. He didn't take all of the pills this time. He is saving the rest for his next round of surgery. Every time I go in the bathroom, I know they are there in the medicine cabinet; I see them often. I think about them, but what I think is, "I'm never going to take another one of those in my life!" That's how I know I've made it.

One day in a Prescription Anonymous support group meeting, we were reading our adaptation of the Twelve Steps, which Alcoholics Anonymous gave us permission to use in our organization. I asked the group what it would take in their lives to be able to move successfully through the Twelve Steps to true recovery. Here's what they said:

1.   Have faith that a solution is possible if you keep searching for it. Adopt an attitude of positive expectations, allowing yourself to be lifted up, to be happy, to grow, to laugh, to cry, to feel all there is to feel.

2.   Learn to forgive yourself: Forgiving yourself means getting back the good that has been lost and moving forward with a new outlook on

life. It means freeing yourself of resentments, embarrassment, guilt, anger and shame. Forgiving yourself means getting another chance, changing your behavior and releasing your past.

3. Take responsibility for at least part of the past so that you have strength over the future. Responsibility means communicating to healthcare providers, pharmacists and dentists that you are a "prescription addict" and/or have dual disorders. Responsibility means no longer blaming others for the mistakes you made.

4. Attend support group meetings frequently to maintain your mental and physical health. Through sharing and listening to others, we learn to be honest with others and ourselves while building self-worth and self-respect.

5. Seek "partners in recovery" and sponsors to ensure their support. The concern, support and input from others are essential to the recovery process. They can identify better than we can our fears and resentments, as well as our addictive behaviors. "Partners in recovery" can be a life link when you need comfort, understanding and structure to minimize relapse.

6. Learn to take charge of your time. Plan your day. Make decisions and choices that serve your recovery and make them early in the day so things don't come at you haphazardly (causing stress) or so you find yourself with nothing to do.

7. Stop looking for magical answers and participate fully in solving your own problems. Magic didn't get you into this and magic isn't going to get you out. You have to work at recovery every day.

8. Live each day with your head held high and as much joy, honesty, trust and serenity as you can.

9. Share with others, as those have before you, the courage, wisdom and serenity you have received through your recovery program.

In the spirit of that last advice, I asked the group to tell me what activities, places or states of mind they seek when they are tempted to relapse. You could ask your support group the same question. Here's what they told me.

> **I love taking time for myself away from distractions to sort things out.**
Solitude gives you a chance to reflect on your day and helps build inner strength and peace. Learning to love solitude means you like being alone

with yourself. If solitude allows you to become depressed or think negative thoughts, you're not ready for it yet. Seek the company of others instead.

> **1 enjoy lighting aromatherapy candles and curling up on the sofa with a good book.**
You should do what makes you feel peaceful when the bad urges or negative feelings hit.

> **1 love to laugh. It makes my heart and stomach feel good!**
Laughter promotes physical and emotional healing. Studies have found that laughter stimulates the immune system by increasing antibodies and lowering cortisol. Call a funny friend or rent a sidesplitting comedy to help raise your spirits.

> **1 enjoy painting and drawing. It helps me express my emotions in a healthy and creative way. It also gives me a sense of accomplishment that is very personal and private.**
Artistic endeavors, like drawing, painting, sculpting, writing poetry, craftwork, dancing and acting, help to release stress and other negative emotions while fighting boredom and providing a sense of pride and accomplishment.

> **Hugs give me a sense of security and calm.**
Touch is very therapeutic and healing. It's intimate and personal. Humans need touch for emotional and spiritual growth. A simple hug can reduce stress and can make someone feel loved and accepted unconditionally. Ask for hugs from your loved ones and tell them to give them liberally. Sometimes, you may have to hug them first.

> **1 enjoy the rejuvenated feeling 1 get after taking a yoga class. Yoga helps me focus on myself. The meditating, stretching and breathing exercises turn off all outside influences.**
There are so many different types of yoga—Hatha yoga, Bhakti, Jnana yoga, Karma yoga, Tantra and others—that you should be able to find one style that is tailored to your needs and goals. Classes can be found in the newspaper, on the Internet, in bookstores, in schools or simply by word of mouth.

> **Falling in love heals me.**
Love is a most powerful tool for healing. Allow yourself to be open to love and freely, unselfishly share it with others. When you open yourself to

love, your spirit blossoms. Love should not be selfish, possessive or jealous. These are neurotic forms of love which are destructive, draining and dangerous to your recovery. When you open yourself up to true love, you open up a world of possibilities.

> **I ask for help from God through prayer.**

Prayer allows you to connect with your higher power (who or whatever it may be), allowing you to ask for forgiveness, offer thanks and ask for healing, courage, wisdom and serenity. When something feels too big for you to handle alone, you can always ask for God's help, because nothing is too big for Him/Her to handle.

> **I've found that when I reward myself for the hard work I've put into staying sober, I reinforce my success and I stick with it.**

Rewards are a great way to congratulate yourself and keep motivated. However, this doesn't mean you should buy out the store (remember that shopping can be a cross-addiction). Limit yourself to one or two small items as a way to say, "Keep up the good work."

> **I call my therapist.**

This is an often-repeated suggestion. If the therapist you have discourages calls when you feel you are in danger of relapsing, get a new therapist about whom you feel good. It is very important to have a positive relationship with your therapist. My therapist (God love her) is a lifeline to peace and understanding without judgement or criticism. She continually encourages me in my addiction recovery and supports my achievements no matter how small or large. She LISTENS where others have not. She guides me as I work through my shame and guilt. She allows me to get my anger out and, if I'm feeling especially vulnerable, she will suggest that I get to a support group meeting or spend time with people I enjoy. If I were close to "using" again, she would strongly suggest that I be admitted into a treatment center for observation until I worked through the reasons for wanting to use drugs again. A good therapist does for you what you can't do for yourself, whenever you need his or her help and until you can stand on your own.

Whether you never relapse or relapse once or a dozen times, all recovering addicts have several goals in common: to live drug-free, to find happiness, to move on with their lives as whole individuals and to leave their pasts behind without resentment or blame. In the beginning, the recovering addict focuses on being alive for just one minute at a time. Then minutes turn into hours, hours into days, days into weeks and finally, months into years of accomplishments and contributions to family, marriage and career. Reaching out for help is the first step, then reaching out again and again if you slip, until finally you are the one to whom people reach out.

A FAMILY DISEASE:

"Please save my wife, because I cannot."

The addict, as long as he is not caught, may think he's not hurting anyone else but himself. However, a person who says her addiction is not hurting her family is engaging in a level of denial. Addiction is a family disease. Addiction affects all members of the family and their behavior—whether it is ignoring or enabling—that allows the addiction to continue.

If you, the reader, are an addict, here is a moving story about what families go through. If you're a family member or friend of an addict, here is an example of others who have suffered in your role.

David, the husband of Shawna, who first described her addiction in chapter 1, tells his story:

David's Story

When I first met Shawna at a church activity in 1991, her beauty, intelligence and charm immediately caught my attention. Shawna was everything that I had been looking for in a woman. We began dating and fell madly in love. One thing that I quickly learned about Shawna was that she sometimes suffered from poor health. She had frequent headaches and fainting spells. In addition, she told me that she had experienced numerous surgeries at a young age—including open heart surgery, back surgery, stomach surgery and gynecological surgery. I thought this was a bit unusual, but knowing about her medical history increased my admiration for her, because she had kept such a positive attitude in the face of adversity. After some careful thought and prayer, I knew in my heart that I loved her enough that her medical problems would not scare me away. Seven months after we met, we were married in Oakland, California. What I did not know at that happy time was that my new wife, the girl of my dreams, was a prescription drug addict.

The first year of our marriage passed and we went through the normal adjustment period that most newly married couples go through. During this time, Shawna continued to have health problems and frequently went to the doctor for a variety of complaints. I was very naïve and never questioned the validity of her problems. The doctor bills were mounting and I began to be concerned. But I never questioned whether or not her problems were real. I trusted her.

One day, out of the blue, Shawna approached me with an anxious look on her pale face. She said that she needed to confess something to me that might cause me to hate her and ruin our marriage. Nervously, I told her to proceed. She said, "You know the medical problems I have been having? Well, I have been faking them...for my entire life." She then added, "And I think I have a problem with taking too many medications." I was devastated. My world would never be the same—and I knew it. She explained that she could not take the pressure of living a lie anymore. She said, "I know I am going to go to hell if I don't make changes in my life."

Not knowing what else to do, I asked her to go speak to our pastor about these problems. He was very kind, but really had no idea how to deal with the issue. As amazing as it now seems, I still was unable to put two and two together. I thought that her admitted problem with faking illness was based on something psychological—perhaps the need for attention—and I didn't connect it with her comment about taking too much medication. I considered the faking of illness to be a much more serious problem.

While she was in counseling with our pastor, I went to the library and began researching psychiatric disorders related to faking illness. I came across some information on a rare disorder known as Munchausen syndrome. This mental illness causes the victim to seek attention from medical personnel and others by feigning sickness. All of the symptoms seemed to fit my wife perfectly. I thought I had discovered her problem. I copied the research and took it to a well-meaning psychiatrist, who met with my wife and confirmed the diagnosis. He informed me that, while there was some hope that she might be cured of this problem, it was unlikely. Most Munchausen patients haunt hospitals, undergoing numerous unnecessary surgeries, for the rest of their lives. Shawna accepted the diagnosis and agreed to go to weekly psychiatric counseling. The doctor also told us that Shawna was suffering from depression and he prescribed antidepressants.

I was so horrified by the Munchausen diagnosis that I completely forgot about my wife's statement that she was taking too much medication. I knew little or nothing about prescription drug abuse. I trusted her doctors and believed that they would never prescribe more medication than she could handle. We did attend one Narcotics Anonymous meeting together, just to find out what the program was all about. I was turned off by the appearance of the addicts and the foul language that was being used in the meeting. I figured these were street-drug users and junkies. My wife and I did not belong among this group of society's outcasts. I now realize the foolishness of this judgment, but, at the time, I wanted nothing to do with these addicts. So we stopped going. I figured that having her admit to the problem with pills was enough. Now that it was out in the open, I believed she would never do it again.

Shawna continued her counseling and seemed to be improving. We did our best to move on and put our marriage and our lives back together again. Our first child, a healthy baby boy, was born in 1993 and brought a great deal of joy to our home.

Despite this wonderful event, something still seemed wrong. Shawna continued to have numerous medical problems, which, of course, made me suspicious. However, despite my concerns, I was unable to prove that any of her problems weren't genuine. She would sometimes have a difficult time getting out of bed to take care of the baby, but I rationalized these incidents away.

Shawna's second pregnancy was a nightmare. She went into early labor and was in and out of the hospital for three months. During this time, she kept pleading for painkillers, because she said the contractions were hurting. Eventually, she gave premature birth to our second child, a little girl, ten weeks before she was due. The baby weighed a little over two pounds. As a father, I cannot begin to describe the terror caused by this event. This is not the way to have a baby. She looked like a little doll— except she had countless tubes and wires attached to her small body. A large machine breathed for her.

Our baby survived, but she spent almost two months in the hospital. Meanwhile, Shawna was getting worse. Her depression came back with a vengeance. The pressure and strain of having a baby in the newborn intensive care unit was unbelievable. The cause of the premature birth was never determined.

One night, Shawna came to me and told me that she was going to kill herself. She said that I would be better off with another wife and that she had a plan to end her life with pills that she had hidden. I tried to reason with her, but she would not listen. She seemed to be in a daze. I immediately took her to the hospital, where they admitted her for severe depression and suicidal ideation. She was confined to the psychiatric ward for a week. During this time, I moved in with my parents who, like angels of mercy, helped take care of my children, so I would not lose my job.

Shawna's depression was so bad that her doctors performed electro-convulsive therapy (ECT) on her. This was a frightening procedure that caused her to lose her short-term memory each time it was done. One time, as she was regaining consciousness, she mumbled to me that she was to blame for our daughter's premature birth. The nurse told her to be quiet and told me not to believe what a person says when they are coming out of anesthesia. This seemed strange, but I believed the nurse.

Shawna was released from the hospital and we all returned home. After a while, she started doing better and desperately wanted to become pregnant again. We consulted our doctor and he told us there was little chance we would have another premature baby and that everything should be fine. So we decided to go ahead and soon conceived another child.

The nightmare returned. Shawna went into early labor and was hospitalized. I could not believe what was happening. Our second baby boy was born eight weeks early. He was very sick, but not as sick as our daughter had been. He was in the intensive care unit for several weeks. Our medical bills were sky high. Each premature birth cost over $80,000. We were struggling financially as a constant wave of medical bills washed up into our mailbox.

Completely worn out from her two premature pregnancies, Shawna again sank into a very deep depression. She was now seeing a psychologist and a psychiatrist. The psychiatrist was giving her some pretty powerful medications—such as Xanax, a benzodiazepine. At the time, I knew nothing about benzodiazepines and was grateful for any help we could get from her doctors.

Then came that fateful night when I came home from work and discovered Shawna in a zombie-like state lying on our couch. She was barely cognizant and was mumbling something that I couldn't understand. I had a feeling that something was terribly wrong. I ran to the cabinet and began going through her medications. I counted over forty missing pills. I could not believe she had taken that much medication. That amount should have *killed the average person. I called Poison Control and they told me her life was in danger. I rushed her to the hospital, where they proceeded to pump her stomach. The next day, she told the doctors she did not remember taking so much medication and that she must have done it by accident. I did not believe her and asked that she be placed in the psychiatric ward for her own protection. In this setting, she finally admitted her prescription drug problem.*

While Shawna was in detox at the hospital, I went to meet with our family doctor. He ran a check on her prescription history (using a state-sponsored database) and discovered that she had been doctor shopping for many years. He told me that she was definitely addicted to painkillers and Xanax. The pieces were all starting to come together. I was relieved to discover that she did not have Munchausen syndrome after all. Many of her fake medical problems in the past could be attributed to drug-seeking behavior. Shawna later admitted that the multiple unnecessary surgeries she had were done just so she could get drugs.

Concerned about the astonishingly high levels of medication that were being prescribed by her psychiatrist, I went to speak with him. I told him about her problem with addiction and he said that he now understood. He said that he would need to taper down the medication, so she would not go into seizures. I trusted him—which turned out to be a huge mistake. At the time, I didn't realize that most physicians have no idea how to handle addiction.

Shawna was released from the hospital and we both decided that she would be better off moving in with her parents (who lived about 180 miles away) until she could put her life back together. I took the kids and moved back in with my parents. This separation was painful, but I figured it was her only chance for success.

Shawna lived with her parents for a couple of months. She attended an outpatient drug abuse program and occasionally came down to visit the children and me. She said that the outpatient program was working and that it was so nice to finally be free of the drugs that had ruled her life. We started making plans to get back together. Then, it happened again.

I was at work one day and I suddenly had a distinct desire to pick up the phone and call Shawna's psychiatrist. His secretary answered and I told her that I wanted to reiterate the fact that Shawna was an addict and that the doctor needed to be careful. The secretary paused for a moment and said, "Shawna just called us for a refill on her Lortab." I practically dropped the phone. Shawna had told me she had not been using Lortab for months. When I asked to speak to the doctor, the secretary told me that he would not talk to me because of laws dealing with patient confidentiality. In fact, I could tell (based on her nervousness) that she realized that she had broken the law by giving me the information about the Lortab. I was furious that the doctor would not speak to me, but I was grateful that the nurse had told me the truth.

I immediately confronted Shawna about the Lortab refill and she started making all kinds of lame excuses. This time, however, I refused to back down. She knew she was caught. She admitted that she had been using while living with her parents. She would have her psychiatrist phone in (long-distance) a variety of prescription drugs. I was at the end of my rope. I told Shawna I was going to leave her and take custody of the children if she did not get her life together immediately. She said she thought she needed to go to inpatient treatment if she was going to have any chance of success. We took her for an evaluation at a government-sponsored inpatient treatment center and they admitted her. I had little faith that, after all the deception, she would be able to turn her life around. Just in case, I looked up the phone number for the county divorce education clerk. This time, I was deadly serious. It was a do-or-die situation. Although I loved Shawna, I honestly had little hope that our marriage could survive this ordeal.

After Shawna went into treatment, I wrote a letter to her psychiatrist (because he wouldn't talk to me), letting him know that I would turn him in to the DEA, his professional board and the state if he continued to prescribe narcotics for my wife. I also threatened to sue him for malpractice because, even though I personally told him that she was an addict, he continued to prescribe addictive medications. I told him I would send him my wife's rehab bill that was rapidly approaching $10,000. My threats appear to have worked. He never prescribed anything for my wife again.

When Shawna went into treatment, I was at the lowest point of my life. I was exhausted and began to feel the cold, icy fingers of depression closing around me. All of my hopes and dreams were gone.

One night, I had a strong feeling that I should drive to my place of worship. It was a cold night and there was snow on the ground. I did not feel worthy to enter, so I stood outside and poured my heart out to God. My prayer went something like this:

"God, I stand before Your house. What kind of a husband am I? My wife has been using drugs for fifteen years and I didn't know it. How can I be so stupid? Why didn't I know? Why didn't you tell me? I once believed *that I could 'fix' my wife's problems, that I had the intellect to diagnose and resolve her condition. I also believed that I could fight her problems with my own strength and wisdom. I have come to You tonight to admit that I have been beaten. This thing called 'addiction' is far too strong for me to deal with. You are the only power in the universe that can slay this beast. I surrender and plead with You to join the battle. Please save my wife, because I cannot."*

In the cold, I could see my own breath and everything around me was silent. Then a feeling of peace and comfort began to warm my heart. I knew God was listening and this matter was now in His hands. I drove home with the feeling that a tremendous burden had been lifted. To this day, I believe God answered my prayer that night.

Shawna was in inpatient treatment for about six weeks. During that time, she experienced terrible withdrawal symptoms—including a seizure that sent her to the hospital. The counselors at the treatment center were able to break through the thick layers of denial that had built up over many years. When she was released, she began attending a day treatment program and went to support meetings every night. The counselors told her that she needed to go to "ninety meetings in ninety days." This was hard on me because it seemed like she was gone so much. However, I understood that it was very important for me not to do anything that would sabotage her recovery efforts.

After several months of being in recovery, Shawna was able to admit that the premature births of our children were probably caused by drug use during the pregnancies. This has been the most difficult issue for both of us to come to terms with. We also discovered that loss of trust is an inevitable consequence of drug abuse. This is something we have really had to work on in our marriage.

I have to admit that, at first, I was terrified to live the rest of my life married to an addict. The counselors told me there was no "cure" for the disease of addiction and that thought scared me. However, I have discovered that living with a recovering addict, as long as they are taking their recovery seriously, isn't much different than living with a non-addict. My wife is clean now and we live a pretty normal life. She needs to go to Narcotics Anonymous meetings a couple times a week, but this is a small price to pay.

In the end, I am especially grateful to God for the miracle that He worked in my family's life. Without His help, I know there would have been no happy ending. I have discovered that God does not give up on any of us very easily. I almost hit the "panic button" with my wife and now I am so glad that I hung in there—even when things got really rough. A marriage is not a trivial thing to break up. God has miraculously restored the love and trust between my wife and me. Together, we now carry His message of hope and freedom to anyone who will listen.

Some people reading David's story, moved as they are by a husband's heartfelt eloquence, may still think, *But I would not have been so naïve. I would have known.* I assure you that many sophisticated and intelligent people, including my husband, have been fooled by the Academy Award-worthy acting of addicts. My husband calls his story "How to Marry an Addict without Really Trying."

How to Marry an Addict without Really Trying: Michael's Story

Where do I begin? When I met Cindy, she was married for the second time. She and my sister were friends and had arranged for the four of us to meet at a comedy club. I distinctly remember telling my sister on the way home how it's too bad that the "good ones" are always taken. She and her husband subsequently moved away and I thought that was the end of it.

Not long after that, Cindy separated from her husband and moved back here and contacted my sister. She came to dinner one night and I knew there was potential for something good between us.

We "dated" for two years, during which time we agreed to take it slowly, as I was unsure about making a long-term commitment and she had two failed marriages behind her. We took the next step by living together to see if we were really compatible. After another year we got engaged and took an additional year to plan the wedding and also get pre-marital counseling at her suggestion. So we knew each other very well by the time we married or so I thought.

Christmas of 1997, when we had been married for five years, we were in Vermont visiting her family. Looking back, I realize that our relationship was in trouble even before that, but I thought it was just part of being married, you know, the "ups and downs." But it became very clear that we were in serious trouble during this holiday. There was a lot of animosity between us and I didn't understand why. We tried to keep our problems from her family, as we didn't want to spoil the holiday for them, but I think they were able to sense something was wrong. Needless to say, that was the worst holiday I have ever experienced.

*We came back home after the holidays and tried to get help through marital counseling. The counselor was female and it seemed to me that she was prejudiced toward my wife's point of view. She made one statement in particular that really spelled out how she felt: "Men love to **fix** things." I remember feeling strong resentment about that annoying comment and particular irritation about the word "fix." I just knew I wasn't going to get equal treatment. So, we stopped seeing this counselor.*

In April 1998, after being together for over nine years and married for five, I got "the phone call." I will always remember the feelings of disbelief I felt when I heard my wife's close friend say Cindy was checking into a mental health institution with "problems." A mental institution! My wife? To say I was shocked is a huge understatement! I was at work trying to provide a nice life for us. I can't remember the details of what I did next—I just remember the feelings of confusion and disbelief. When did this happen? What caused it? How could I not have known?

I soon learned that she had become addicted to prescription drugs long before I met her. Imagine how it feels to find out the person who has been your partner for almost ten years has been under the influence of one medication or another the whole time and you never saw her "straight!" I said I was naïve, but even now it is difficult to accept my "blindness" to it.

As it happened, there was a workshop being held at the treatment facility the week following her admittance. Of course, I decided to take a few days off from work and attend some sessions to try and learn what was going on and how I could help.

I can remember how absurd the idea of Cindy's addiction seemed to me at the time. After all, there were people "out there" who had lost loved ones, some who were living (or existing) in boxes on the street and so many other tragic stories. Compared to that, my wife (I thought) had no right to have emotional problems. She was well provided for materially, had a devoted husband, two families who loved and cared about her and many friends...she had so much more than so many other people! This was my view. Now, although there is still a certain amount of logic there, I can better see the flaws in my thinking, because of the eye-opening education and experience I have received since that time.

*My very presence at the workshop was a result of my thinking I could **fix** my wife's problems. There was that word again. During the workshop, several people told me in group sessions that I couldn't fix my wife's problems and I was wrong for trying. Of course, I responded very defensively. After all, isn't that what you do when you care about someone? You do* *what you can to fix her problem. It made no sense to let her flounder on her own, if there was something I could do to help. I now refer to that time in my life as the "Before the Light Came on" or "Before I Got it" period. Looking back from where I am now, I can still remember what it felt like— the confusion and frustration of it all. I consider this to be a positive thing, as it helps me remember what it took to "get it" or "for the light to come on." It took a long recovery process for me as well as for Cindy.*

During her stay in the health facility, I had the unenviable task of informing both our families, as it was a serious situation and I thought they should know at least something about it. The question was just how much to tell them and how much they would understand. I knew how they might respond, as I had just gone through the same shock and denial myself. There was no way for them to speak to her while she was in treatment and, besides, she told me she didn't want to speak to anyone during that time anyway. I did the best I could and they all showed the proper concern for her and for me. I told them I would try to keep them informed.

After Cindy was released, she felt better, but we knew we had a long road ahead of us. We spent the rest of the year trying to cope with our situation, but it wasn't going very well. She kept telling me that I needed to attend a program of my own if it was going to work for us. I still didn't "get it," so I didn't think I needed help. I agreed to try an Al Anon meeting, but only to help her—I was in denial and still trying to fix things. After a few weeks of listening to women talk about their drunk, abusive husbands, I decided that I was not benefiting from the meetings, so I stopped going. My quitting didn't help the situation between Cindy and me, which continued to deteriorate.

Cindy kept insisting that I needed a recovery program of my own, so I agreed to try a different Al Anon meeting at a different location. What a difference from the previous ones I had attended! Right from the start, the members said things I could relate to, including the fact that you have to try several different meetings to find the "right" one for you. I knew then that I had found the right place, but I also knew it was going to take some time for me to feel comfortable enough to open up and share my personal life with a group of strangers. The amazing thing was that almost everyone who spoke sounded like me, which made it much easier to share with them. This was the beginning of a turning point for me, but it wasn't enough yet to turn our situation around.

What I didn't know is that breaking the addiction to drugs is even harder on relationships than the addiction itself. A side effect of giving up drugs is depression and my wife was feeling it big time! She relapsed on the day before Thanksgiving. To make a long story short, this relapse involved the police, an ambulance, another one of those dreaded phone calls to me and her ending up back in the treatment facility on suicide watch. I didn't feel there was much to be thankful for that Thanksgiving.

Within a month, Cindy informed me that she needed to leave home to help her focus on her recovery. My initial reaction to this was strong opposition. First, I didn't believe she could solve this problem by running away from it. Second, and more importantly, I believed that a couple should work on their problems together. Although I had started my recovery and we had been going to individual counseling, I still wasn't able to let go of my previous way of thinking—the light bulb was still off!

I knew I couldn't prevent her from leaving and, as it turned out, it was the best thing she could have done for both of us. Here she was—the so-called "sick one"—but she was smarter than I was in making that decision. She had begun her recovery and she was learning her recovery had to come first—without it, there could be nothing else!

We had been "butting heads" on a daily basis, usually about trivial matters, but we both knew there was an underlying cause. The most important benefit of her absence was that I had so much time to digest all that had transpired and absorb the information I had received regarding my part in our situation. The light bulb began flickering. I was starting to get it!

The true test of my new awareness came when Cindy told me she was going to file for divorce. I knew I had to "let go" if we were going to make it. I also knew that, as much as it hurt and would for some time, I would survive—my Higher Power would see to that! That's when our miracle happened. The light bulb turned on and my "getting it" coincided with "letting go." I don't know if she sensed the change in my outlook or was getting a clearer picture of herself, but, after five months of separation, she asked if she could come home. That is worthy of being called a miracle—at least to me!

We were both a little apprehensive at first, which seems natural after what we had been through. But we both knew this time it would be different. We were and are both in recovery. She has her program, I have my program and we have our program. That's not to say we don't have setbacks. Being in recovery does not make you stop being human beings, which means that human nature can and will continue to cause conflict between individuals. Being in recovery also means it is a lifelong journey, without ending, which means you are never "cured." It means you—both the user and the code-pendent or enabler—have the tools to live a good life by recognizing the disease of addiction and what it is capable of and to take the steps neces-sary to keep it in check. It really isn't difficult once your "light bulb" comes on or you "get it." Any way you want to put it, it just means altering your lifestyle to live your life in a positive way. It's really just that simple, but not to be confused with easy! You become part of a new family with your partners in recovery, from whom you gain strength by knowing there are others like you. You, in turn, get to give back by showing others the same thing.

I cannot emphasize enough the pride I feel for my wife, myself and all of the people who are in recovery with us and for the courage and commitment it took to get us from where we were to where we are. The program really works, but it works a little bit differently for each of us and it only works for you if you are willing to work for it!

In both of these stories, Shawna's husband and my husband reached turning points when they finally "let go" and stopped trying to fix things themselves. This is what we in Prescription Anonymous and other addiction groups mean by "Let go and let God."

Another person in the family who suffers greatly is the child of an addict. Marjorie was a mother addicted to prescription drugs. What happened to her was bad enough, but an additional tragedy was that the children in her family thought their unhealthy family dynamics represented normal family life. Her children grew up without normal social skills, using deceit to avoid being close to other people. Her story shows how deeply the illness of addic-tion affects the entire family. Her son Brandon relates how the family coped with his mother's addiction.

Brandon's Story

My mom's addiction started early in her life. When she was twelve years old, her parents divorced and her grandmother gave her sleeping pills to help her rest. It was the 1950s and America was in the era of Mother's Little Helper, in which doctors, delighted with a new array of pharmaceuticals designed for stress disorders and panic attacks, were handing out serious mood elevators to depressed patients like candy. My mother, like other children in this era, grew up in a pill happy environ-ment. No one could foresee the effects these pills would have on families for generations to come. By the time I was born, my mom had a bent for pills, often in combination with alcohol, that would take the edge off her mounting responsibilities. Her marriage to my dad during that time was all fun and games. They had friends, a nice house, my newborn sister and myself. Life for my mom was consistent. She was the model housewife. My dad was an up-and-coming salesman who went to school at night to secure a bright future. The first danger signs I remember coincided with a move to the country. Big parties on weekends, which were fun for all us kids, usually ended with my mom having to be put to bed. The first glimpses into the vortex of disaster were those moments of uncertainty, not knowing the problem or why Mom was acting so funny. And so it went year after year—not understanding what was really going on—until the birth of my baby brother, when I saw the intensity of her illness growing. My dad by now was on the road a lot with his job, so the job of "watching Mom" became a normal thing for me and my sister. We learned the art of trickery to keep my mom out of trouble and her problem a secret from the outside world: we hid the pills, watered down or poured out all liquors and, most importantly, hid the car keys. Dad's wrath for letting her drive the car away was harsh, so we were very efficient at our job. Protecting the image of the family became the status quo. I was a master liar by age ten. Concocting stories to elude friends and teachers when she didn't come to pick me up from school is one example of the nightmare that was our normal family routine.

Meanwhile, the country doctor, who essentially was her dealer, didn't read the signs or maybe he did and it was easier to look the other way. Besides, he probably had a new car from all the money that my dad paid trying to make mom well. It was like everybody knew about Mom, but didn't know what to do except give her a different kind of pill.

Therapy seemed logical, but brought out more destructive patterns. The more psychiatrists pried into the hurt resulting from the divorce of Mom's parents, the more she would shut the door and hide in her little, inner world of hurt where she used the one and only thing that would take all the pain away—PILLS!

Mom learned to speak "The Language" which enabled her to get any kind of pill. One memory comes to mind: When I was with my mom at the doctor's office and she explained her symptoms, the doctor proceeded to pull out a pill book that looked like the kind of tablet that Charleston Heston had in his role of Moses. I'd never seen anything so big in my life. And when he opened it up, it was nothing but pages and pages of colorful rows and rows of pills. The doctor would flip through the pages, all the while listening to my mom and, finally, like pinning the tail on the donkey, he would point to a specific pill and say, "Let's try this one!"

It was absurd to me that she even bothered visiting a doctor to get more pills. She already had a mini pharmaceutical company in our kitchen cabinets. Every time we opened a cabinet door to find some food, a small, caramel colored bottle with a white childproof cap would come tumbling out.

The real challenge came with my years as an adolescent male, the whole thing of being a young buck. Hell, I was forced to grow up so fast that I felt like a twenty-five-year-old in a fourteen-year-old body. I had seen things no child should ever see and it had made me skeptical of those who really did seem to care about my family and me. The ability to enjoy my youth was tainted with dread. I was always wondering if bringing home new friends wouldn't turn out to be like a scene from the Addams Family. Therefore the desire to make friends was hampered and I started to hide within a shell of books and adolescent fantasy.

By this time, the relationship that had seemed somewhat normal between mom and dad began to deteriorate. My dad's frustration and inexperience dealing with emotions that come from the heart fed the fire. He started to distance himself from her and us. Physical fights between them were becoming more and more frequent. Then we had to lie to cover up the reason for my mom's wearing sunglasses around the house. Craziness erupted in the middle of the night as my mom fought off the demons in her sleep. Every day my mom had a new problem and every day was a battle to hide whatever we thought was the problem. A never-ending series of cyclonic episodes destroyed our home life. The peaks and valleys of alternating good times and bad times were slowly killing a little part of all our hearts. We were learning about the true definition of addiction and we didn't even know the word addiction. We learned to distance ourselves and create modes of operation that were escape mechanisms and temporary ploys of entertainment, which took us away from the reality of our lives, where things could turn on a dime.

My out, my escape, came with a scholarship to college. Eager to experience a new life, I hoped that the tumult that filled my home would disappear and I would have a chance to have a normal life. What I soon realized was the modes of living at home were far less cruel than the ones that awaited me in the real world. I had spent so much time at home absorbed with Mom that I hadn't learned the social skills needed to protect myself. Instead, I had learned a set of skills that were now inappropriate.

Learning quickly how people operate was a new hobby—watching after my mom had chiseled me into a master of details—and I was a virtuoso of deceit. College soon became a snap. I made it through without people really knowing me or my past. This also relieved me from true responsibility in the sense that in order to have true friends, I concluded, you have to take on a lot of their baggage, help them, pamper them, give them a lot of time and effort. Frankly, I didn't have the time or heart for others.

I was relieved to no longer have the responsibility of dealing with my mother. My relationship with her was reduced to a random series of phone calls. I would sit and listen to her idle chatter, tell her how much I loved her and say goodbye. I had become hardened and didn't want to deal with all her problems.

I had become self-absorbed, not really caring about anyone, including my first wife—which is a shame, because she really tried to understand my moods. I went though my life intensely wanting to be part of something; however, I never really made an effort to be part of anything. It was a debilitating circle. I went through my life in a series of near successes, never grabbing the brass ring, but learning a lot of hard lessons along the way.

My second chance came with meeting the person who would help me heal. My second wife took the time to listen and not judge. She and my mom bonded immediately with the birth of my first child. And it looked like things were finally changing. Mom had become fairly stable. There was still the occasional binge, but everyday life had started to change when she began giving her time to teach Sunday school at a local Unity Church. Her search for something more in life was finally being realized. What she was so intently looking for had been there, right in front of her face. She was fighting addiction with new confidence and renewed vision. Just as my mom had finally turned toward the light, it was as if she decided she had endured enough and, without warning, died in her sleep at the age of fifty-four.

My mom is dead and it had everything to do with what she had put into her body over the years. There is no one single person to blame, although I have tried to find one. The only person who could have changed the story was my mother herself.

I will always be angry that my mom won't be here to see my family grow and I will always be angry that she wasn't strong enough to say no to prescription drug abuse. I will always be angry with the doctors who never really tried to cure her, but instead tried out another medicine du jour. *I will always miss the beautiful smile that welcomed me into this world. I am angry that I will never again be able to say, "I love you," to her face and hug her and tell her how proud I am that she finally found some relief from the talons of her addiction. It is too late.*

"Too late" are the saddest words. Could Brandon's story of his mother Marjorie's addiction and death have been changed? Maybe. Truthfully, we'll never know. And that is one of the hardest parts of "too late"—the finality of death, not getting the chance to say all the things you wanted to say and not knowing what the future might have held if things turned out differently. But such a tragedy did not have to be.

The next chapter illustrates how families—the addict and his or her loved ones—can recognize addiction, intervene, support and participate in recovery so that their stories do not end like Brandon's and Marjorie's.

RECOVERY AND THE FAMILY:
"We had become strangers overnight."

Whole families fall into denial when one member is addicted to prescription drugs. Usually it's the addict's spouse who has to deal most intimately with the addiction. Yet that person likely knows little or nothing about the signs of addiction. Even though he or she may be closest to the addicted individual, a spouse often doesn't see what is happening or is in denial about it. "My wife couldn't be addicted to prescription drugs or over-the-counter medicines, she would know better," the unsuspecting husband might say.

At the same time, the addict lives in denial when it comes to the effects addiction has on family and loved ones. "I never realized the pain and suffering I caused my family. Once my addiction to pills took over my life, I never thought I was hurting anyone else. I was the sick one, what effect could this have on them?" So says Ellen, a recovering addict recalling her denial.

Former first lady Betty Ford, who became addicted to pain pills following surgery and who founded the Betty Ford Clinic after her recovery, calls prescription addiction "a hidden epidemic." Abuse, she said, "is swept under the rug by the prescription addict and by desperate families and friends. They can't accept the reality of a mother or aunt or sister who may be abusing pills or is addicted to pills and they simply don't know what to do about it."[1]

If the addict can hide his addiction from himself, he can hide it from others. It takes a person who is aware of the possibility of addiction to look at the signs and recognize them.

Here are some warning signals that might indicate that a loved one has an addiction problem.

The person:
> Has a substantial increase in visits to doctors and dentists.
> Schedules surgeries that may not be necessary.
> Has an unexplained increase in medical bills.
> Frequently cancels plans with friends or family.
> Has a difficult time on the job or is losing a lot of time from work.
> Doesn't look you in the eyes while talking.
> Has a range of physical symptoms, for example, is hyperactive; has quick weight loss or gain; is bloated or flushed.
> Sometimes will call someone to "just talk," but can't remember the conversation the next day.
> Keeps prescription pills handy at all times and offers them freely to friends.
> Roams around the house lethargically and without purpose.
> Is moody, irritable or restless; sleep patterns change.
> Spends most of his time alone and screens phone calls.
> Has money problems, borrows cash and runs up charges on her credit cards.
> Acts contrary to his values, such as stealing, lying and having extra-marital affairs.

Even when family members or friends do begin to get the picture, not knowing how to help, they often continue the behavior of denial and, consequently, enable the addict. A family member or colleague may say, "Don't you think she's acting peculiar?" or "I know for a fact she's not supposed to be taking so many of those...."

Then someone else says, "Have you talked to her?"

And the first person replies, "You know you can't talk to her, she'll just get angry and say...," "Besides, it's not my place" or "I don't want to ruin Christmas...."

Spouses in particular often feel responsible for their partners' addictions just as parents feel responsible for the addictions of their children. Families feel a need to keep the addiction a secret out of shame, fear of criticism, pride, a desire to protect the addict and fear of financial consequences. While trying to keep this secret, family members often become controlling and rigid, yet at the same time they often feel powerless, hopeless and depressed. It is quite common for the family to become as disabled by the addiction as the addicted person does.

What's more, family members may be playing into the disorder, a behavior known as "enabling." Enabling is any act that interferes with the natural consequences of destructive behavior. Although enabling is born out of caring, love and concern for the addict (as well as self-protection), it perpetuates the disorder by reinforcing the addict's behavior and keeping an individual from recognizing his or her problem and getting help.

Examples of enabling:
> Making excuses to cover behavior. For instance, a husband might call his wife's office and say she is ill, when she is actually incapacitated by drug misuse.
> Pretending not to notice destructive behavior.
> Consoling the addicted loved one by blaming others for the problem.
> Giving assurances that the behavior is normal.
> Agreeing that others are wrong to worry.
> Keeping silent ("speak no evil, hear no evil, see no evil").

Now an adult, Matthew, the child of an addict recalls, "As far back as I can remember I have always covered up for my father, looking the other way. I always looked up to my father. How could I confront him with my suspicions that he was abusing his pills?"

Recognizing an addiction, but failing to act against it, going along with it or accommodating it is a form of denial. It enables the addictive behavior. I am not blaming those who enable addiction, certainly not children. Enabling is a normal reaction. People naturally think, "What can I do? I don't know how to fix this." Not enabling—that is, letting the addict feel the natural consequences of his actions—may mean the addict will lose his job or worse and the spouse and children may suffer from such a disaster as much or more than the addict.

Joe, the husband of an addict, says, "I know I am enabling her when I make excuses to her boss so she won't lose her job. But the mortgage is based on both our incomes and we just can't do without it right now."

Beth now realizes she was enabling her husband's addiction when she took a job she didn't want just to earn more money so he didn't have to work. "At the time, he couldn't work. Who would hire him? He couldn't pass a drug test. What choice did I have?"

It's clear that enablers are often in just as much of a bind as the addict. It seems difficult or impossible for both to bring an end to the problem.

However, it is important to realize that the self-protective behavior of the enabler allows an individual to continue his or her addiction without severe consequences. Which brings up The Big Question: What will you do down the road if the addiction continues? Divorce? Kick the person out? Suffer as you do now? Bury him or her? Are those long-term consequences worse than the immediate consequences you would face if you stopped enabling and let nature take its course?

When something happens to force the issue of addiction out into the open or when an individual takes the brave step of admitting the problem and seeking help, the rest of the family is suddenly thrust into a struggle as threatening as if they had fallen into the strong current of a roaring river. If you are suspicious or aware of the plight of a loved one who has not sought help, you may be trying to come up with a plan of assistance before you are suddenly thrown into the icy water. I support you in your desire to intervene.

If there are prescription bottles and over-the-counter medicines that the person you are concerned about uses, copy all the doses, directions, refill information, prescribing doctor, etc. for each bottle and count the pills in each one. Keep a record of the rate at which they disappear and do the same for any additional bottles that show up. These may not be all the pills the person is using, but you may be able to record a pattern of abuse for the ones you see. Having the facts will help you bring the person out of denial. But don't confront the addicted individual until you have a plan.

Sometimes, a well-planned family "intervention" can help a person examine her life and decide that she does need help. While even the best intervention offers no guarantee, there is a better chance of getting positive results from an intervention if the entire family supports it. Enlist the help of sympathetic family members, best friends and even a supportive boss who is aware of the problem. Ask them to join you, but do not try to persuade someone who is unwilling. Ask everyone involved to read about addiction and recovery. You could hand them this book. You could ask them to go to a meeting of Al Anon, the Alcoholics Anonymous support group for family members.

An intervention requires planning on the parts of all the people involved. Ideally, you would be able to ask a therapist or pastor with inter-vention experience and training to help you design the intervention and to be present to guide you through the process. After all, when those involved meet to plan the intervention, things may not go smoothly. One relative or friend may blame another. They may say: "You should have seen this and stopped it; you were the one who was with her every day" or "This problem comes from your side of the family." Others may complain about having to be involved, asking you why you can't stop this nonsense by yourself. A trained therapist can help bring people together and teach them how to be respectful of one another and of the person you are trying to help. An intervention counselor can set up guidelines and help each person plan his or her part of the script. There should be at least one practice session with the counselor. Anyone who cannot join in respectfully or follow the rules must be asked to excuse him or herself. More about formal interventions guided by professionals can be found at www.intervention.com. Whether or not you have a professional interventionist to guide you, do not schedule an intervention until you have a treatment plan in place.

Collect information about professional assessment and available treatment centers now. Call and ask about admission policies, costs and insurance issues. Get recommendations for therapists with training and experience in addiction. As you gather this information, keep it and this book handy for the moment when you need them.

If the person you are trying to help observes your efforts to collect information, you will likely be propelled a little faster into confrontation, which may mean having an intervention a bit before you are ready. Confrontation occurring sooner than you planned is no reason for panic. If it happens, it happens. Whether you choose the timing or not, if you have gathered all the information and kept it handy, you are more prepared for the confrontation than you may realize. If necessary, let the addict rage. At some level, she knows the truth and she knows things can't go on the way they have been.

Are you scared? Of course. Do you hesitate? Naturally.

Just remember this: If a loved one or friend were sick with a physical disease, you'd do everything you could to help, wouldn't you? In fact, prescription addiction is a medically proven physical disease just like diabetes, cancer and heart disease—and it's just as life-threatening if untreated. One difference is that your beloved addict may be resisting your efforts. But this is when he needs your help the most. The silent cry you cannot hear says, "I need you to do for me what I can't do for myself."

By confronting a loved one and telling him in a caring manner how his behavior has affected his family and friends, you may be able to break through the wall of denial and greatly increase the likelihood that he will get professional help. Regardless of the outcome, the person with the disease will never be able to engage in the unacceptable behavior in the same way again knowing you know. Once everything is out in the open, the situation is changed forever. If you're concerned, talk now. If you wait, more harm will come to your loved one.

If you are searching for the words to get started, borrow one of the following:

> Nancy, we love you very much. But we have noticed a change in your personality and you've been isolating yourself from everyone. We're worried about you. We know you have been filling a number of prescriptions lately, but you don't appear to be sick. We want to help you in any way we can if you'll let us.
> Gail, I'm not a professional, so I can't tell if you have a problem. But I can see that something is affecting you. Remember the wedding we all went to where you cried uncontrollably at the table? Or the numerous times you have forgotten conversations we had only days before? You might want to have a professional assessment done to find out just what the problem may be, whether emotional or physical. I know the names of some good professionals I'd be happy to share.
> Steven, you're my best friend and I care about what's been happening to you. I've noticed for a while now that you're moody and you look depressed. I've noticed you're taking more pain pills than instructed. You've always been there for me when I had a problem, so I would like to help you, if I can.
> Seth, I can only go by what I see. I do know something is affecting you that has me worried. Remember the night you called me at 2:00 A.M. and you didn't remember the next day? Or the day you yelled at the waitress for not refilling your water glass? You used to not act out this way; you were always in control of everything. You might want to seek help from a professional, someone who can help you through whatever is going on. I'll even make an appointment and take you myself if you will let me.

Once the ice is broken and the confrontation has been gently begun, add progressive pressure. Here's how:

1. Confront the addicted person with your suspicions in a calm, loving and caring manner, saying, "I have a concern...." Use "I" phrases such as "I noticed" or "I'm worried" about the incident instead of "you"

phrases: "You never take pills as directed." A person can't argue with your feelings.

2. Don't blame, criticize or be judgmental. You're intervening because you care, not to make her see how bad she is.

3. Don't worry if you don't say things perfectly. The most important thing is to express your concern in a caring and honest way with an open mind.

4. Be specific. Bring up incidents such as "When I saw you take more pills than instructed this morning at breakfast..." or "I heard you make appointments with two different doctors on the same day for the same complaint" or whatever evidence of abuse you have personally witnessed.

5. Be prepared for the addict to deny that he or she has a problem with prescription or over-the-counter medicine addiction. This is one of the unfortunate symptoms of this disease. Don't take it personally.

6. Talk about the effects of pill misuse on whatever the addict cares about most: this could be his children, spouse, family, looks or job. He very well may not be concerned about himself right now, but may care deeply about his children or marriage; or he may not care about his health, but is very appearance-conscious. In fact, if you are the spouse and you have made up your mind that you will leave the marriage and take the children if the addict doesn't seek treatment, tell him that. Or if you are the boss and you know you must fire this employee unless she recovers fast, now is the time for the ultimatum. Don't deliver it in anger, just state the consequences of a failure to seek treatment. Tell him, "I love you, but this behavior has to end" or "I value you as an employee, but I can't risk the consequences of keeping you." Or, in extreme cases, "I will call the police if you do not permit me to drive you to a treatment center." If the addicted person refuses to seek help, make sure you follow through with the consequences so that he or she will know just how serious you are.

7. A prescription addict will sometimes be hesitant to enter a treatment center or fear going to support group meetings because, on top of feeling guilty, ashamed, angry and embarrassed, she also feels guilty about taking time for herself and spending less time with her children, on her job or taking care of other personal responsibilities. Remind her that most treatment programs are only a few weeks and that support group meetings are only an hour. By taking time to

recover and get healthy, she will actually be more available to her family and other duties. Remind her that focusing on herself for the first time in a long time is not only okay, it's a necessity.

8. If and when the addict agrees to go to a treatment center, offer to sit with her while she makes the arrangements. Offer to drive her to a treatment center or therapist who will decide whether the addict needs outpatient or residential care. Reassure her over and over that she is doing the right thing. Tell her how supportive you will be and stay with her while she is being assessed.

9. If the addict is impaired, suicidal, dangerous or ill, call 911. Emergency personnel will judge whether to send an ambulance or police if necessary to take him to a hospital or other appropriate facility. A mental health facility is required by law in most states to hold a person for seventy-two hours for evaluation to determine if the afflicted person is suicidal or a danger to himself or others.

Regardless of the outcome of your intervention and offering of support, you as a spouse, friend or family member are likely to feel tremendous relief in the knowledge that you have done all you can do to help your loved one and yourself. Exposing the problem means you will never again have to pretend that nothing was wrong.

Telling the Children

In families with children living at home, a parent going into treatment requires explanation and comforting. Ideally, both parents discuss between themselves what they will tell the children. Talking to your own children about going away for treatment requires an understanding of their maturity level and their needs. Decide what you are comfortable telling them as long as it's truthful and something they will be able to handle. Then bring it up together in a family meeting so everyone will know what has been said and how everyone reacted. This sharing of information openly tells the children that this is not a family secret they must hide and never talk about. Let them know you all are dealing with the problem together, each helping the other out.

What you tell the children should have four parts: If you are the addicted parent, tell the children first that you have a problem, second, that you are going to get help for it and third, that you will get better. Fourth, ask them if they have any questions about the situation and answer them honestly.

Throughout the four explanations and forever after, talk to your children honestly. Don't give them false information about your problem that will keep them from understanding your addiction. Later, when they may want to understand the whole picture more clearly, they will need to be able to rely on the earlier information given to them. When you feel you must withhold information, because the children will not be able to understand or deal well with the particulars due to their age or level of maturity, generalize rather than give misinformation. For example, it is all right to tell a young child that you are sick and are going to a hospital, because addiction is an illness. You may also say you feel sad rather than depressed, because this concept will be better understood. You might explain to an older child that you are having trouble giving up painkillers and that these medications are not good for you, so you are going to go to a special hospital where you can be more comfortable learning to give them up. With an older child, you might tell him you have been feeling very depressed, also, if that is the case. People who are afraid it will be harmful for a child to know about a drug addiction should be aware that giving a good example about facing and curing addiction may prove to be a very important lesson for that child. It will teach him to be wary of drugs, to know drugs can cause problems and to know that it is good to take charge and seek help for his own problems in the future.

Reassure children that the treatment you are seeking will be very helpful and that they, along with the whole family, will benefit from your becoming well again. "I won't seem so sad anymore and we will have more fun together," you could say. Explain to older children about sobriety and how you will work hard to resist temptation.

Ask the children if they have questions. The questions they ask will give you insight into how much they understand, about how they feel and about what else to tell them.

As I said, having the type of conversations discussed are ideal. However, the departure for a treatment center or even jail does not always allow such a measured approach. Moreover, the addicted person may be incapable of talking calmly and reassuringly to his or her children. In that case, it is best that the other parent or caregiver say these things on behalf of the parent who is going for treatment. The conversation should follow the same four steps. First, you could calmly say that Mom or Dad has a problem with pills and is going away to seek help. Second, reassure the children that their parent will get better and be a better parent when he or she returns. Next, promise your attention and support during this time. Finally, invite the children to ask questions for you to answer honestly and as fully as is appropriate for their level of understanding.

You're In This Together

Just as the family's denial shadows the addict's denial, so does family chaos mirror the chaos in the addict's life when she first admits the problem and seeks help. For every step the addict takes, from denial on, there is a family counterpart as addict and family struggle toward recovery together.

During treatment by choice, persuasion or force, the addict will change for the better. If you are a family member, what you may be less prepared for is that you also will change. If you had a part in the addict's life before, you will have a changed role in his life from now on. We live through personal interactions and if one person behaves differently, the other will have to change. If you confronted your loved one about his addiction, he had to react. When he comes home sober, you may find you are living with a stranger. The whole family is in recovery now.

That is why I strongly recommend that everyone in the family go to an Al Anon support group meeting or the family support group of any addiction organization. Also, I strongly urge spouses of addicts to get therapy, both individual and couple's counseling.

Remember Pat's story in the first chapter of this book? Pat couldn't deal with the changes necessary when her alcoholic husband went into treatment. Remember my husband Michael, who discovered that he had a lot to learn in therapy and Al-Anon? Remember, too, that he had to try more than one group before he found a good fit? Keep in mind the lessons Michael, Pat and others have learned when you are going through this ordeal and try to avoid making the same mistakes they did.

Couples and family members from an Al-Anon group have suggested these helpful hints for recovering addicts and their partners.

DOs AND DON'Ts IN RECOVERY

DOs

> Do learn as much as you can about prescription addiction as well as other dual diagnoses (i.e. depression, anxiety, suicidal tendencies and cross-addictions such as gambling.)
> Do go to couple's therapy, both private counseling and individual support groups for feedback from others who have been there.
> Do talk to others in the prescription addict's family, like her parents and siblings and even her closest friends, to keep them updated if the addict can't bear to talk with them herself. Ease the stress by communicating with them until the addict can face these people. She should not be rushed or pushed. She will know when she is ready.

> Do go to the pharmacy to fill and refill prescriptions in the beginning (a few weeks to a month) of recovery. Make arrangements for someone other than the recovering addict—a neighbor, therapist or friend—to dispense the medications until you and the addict feel he can manage them without temptation.
> Do listen, listen, listen to your loved one in recovery without interruption. Don't just hear the words, absorb them.
> Do freely communicate your feelings.
> Do allow others to express opinions different from yours. Keep an open mind.
> Do have a lot of patience with your loved one's mood swings, irritability and sudden unexplained crying.
> Do make time to do fun things together again. It may have been a while.
> Do give constant reassurance that everything will be okay and that you will work together on getting through this time of crisis. Make the recovering addict feel less alone in his own home. After a few months pass, you both will no longer feel like you are walking on eggshells.
> Do remember hugs, kisses and romance. Re-ignite the romance. It's a brand new beginning, make the most of it! Changing the way you live doesn't mean forgetting what it was like to be happy with each other.

DON'Ts
> Don't blame each other for all the problems now being faced. Both of you are feeling hurt enough already. Don't try to figure out "how we got into this mess" but "how we are going to get out of this mess together."
> Don't make judgements or criticize each other. Think before you speak.
> Don't keep medicines—yours or your spouse's—out in the open for easy access for a month or until the addict can manage his medications alone.
> Don't keep alcohol in the house or allow others to drink around the addict until she feels that it is no longer a trigger or temptation.
> Don't leave your loved one alone if you suspect that she is not feeling "safe" from the temptation to misuse. Ask a friend or family member to stay with her for a while when you are out, until your partner says she's ready to be alone.

> Don't close yourself off from the problem. Isolating yourself will only stop all communication. The addict needs all your support and understanding now more than ever.

The impact family and friends can have on the addict's success—or failure—in recovery should not be underestimated. Shawna, whose story appears in several places in this book, relates a touching anecdote of what family support did for her. After she pretended to be in recovery, she secretly continued using pills. When her husband found out, he told his mother what Shawna was doing. Shawna's in-laws immediately came to the young couple's home to help. This is what happened next, as Shawna remembers it:

My mother-in-law came into my room and rubbed my back as I sobbed and held myself in the fetal position on the bed. She kept telling me how much she loved me and that she would do whatever it took to get me well. She then said, "Turn around and look at me, Sweetie." I turned around, my face drenched with tears and shame, and I looked at her and said, "How can you still love me after all that I've done to you, your son and your family?" She replied, "You are my Shawna." I knew right then that I was not going to have to endure this alone.

Shawna learned a great deal about the benefits of supportive loved ones during her difficult struggle to end her dependence on prescription drugs. She urges family and friends of addicts in recovery to learn from her story and heed her advice:

As a family member or friend, please be your loved one's greatest support system. What he or she is going through is pure and utter hell. You must be there for her or him, without enabling addictive behavior. I hated my husband and family at the time for bringing my secret out in the open and forcing me to get help, but I will be eternally grateful for their firm, unwavering support and love.

THE PEACE OF RECOVERY:
"I look back and see where I was before and I cry tears of joy."

You think you've made it. But...how can you be sure? First, you are never free from danger and you will always be in recovery. You are never finished because you can always go back to your old ways and you can always grow more. Still, there are signs of achievement and feelings of serenity that mark real recovery.

You know you've made it when...

> You believe in yourself because you have just succeeded at something very, very difficult where failure had always prevailed before.
> The good times have finally outweighed the bad, whereas before bad was all you knew.
> You and your spouse or partner have learned to listen with your hearts every day to better understand each other's needs.
> You have made amends with those whom you hurt during your illness and you feel the weight of guilt lifted from your shoulders as relationships begin to heal.
> You have resolved feelings of guilt and shame.
> You have developed a meaningful life.
> You have rediscovered pleasure and satisfaction in your day-to-day activities.
> You have restored positive values and spiritual beliefs.
> You are able to live in peace with yourself even through unsolved problems. You have found self-soothing techniques other than drugs and you are making healthy solutions with a clear mind.

> Concern for yourself lessens as you gain interest in others.
> You intuitively handle situations that used to baffle you.
> You have begun to understand the words, "peace of mind."

Here is a different kind of "test" for recovery. It asks you to look both within and without and assess yourself at this moment. How many positive changes do you see in your condition now? The changes you can check off are a measure of your progress. The changes you cannot currently check off are benefits you will soon observe on your road to recovery.

How many changes do you see?

- I'm feeling healthier again
- My headaches are less frequent
- Physical pains are less frequent
- My stomach doesn't ache
- My stomach is less upset
- Chest pressure is going away
- I don't cry as often
- I find myself smiling more often
- My blood pressure has returned to normal
- I can see clearly; my eyes are focused
- I'm eating normally, healthier
- I'm less anxious or nervous
- My sense of humor has returned
- I feel good about my accom- plishments and goals
- I feel I can be honest with myself and others
- I can hold onto a job
- I don't feel violent anymore
- My creativity has returned
- I have improved communica- tions
- I feel loved and wanted
- I feel grateful for my recovery
- My life is getting better and better
- I feel I can help others in need
- I don't get as angry as I used to
- Concentration has improved
- Sex has improved
- I think more clearly
- It feels good to not want to abuse pills anymore
- I get to work on time
- I get more compliments from others
- I physically look better
- I can concentrate better
- I feel like a winner
- I feel organized
- I feel less guilty about my past behavior
- I have learned to trust myself
- I have learned to forgive myself
- I want to live
- I have a positive attitude
- I can feel comfortable around people
- I feel less anxious with my family
- I have made amends with my family
- My love relationships have improved

Here are some voices of inspiration from people who have been through the worst to find life again in their souls. These people have "arrived."

> *I have found harmony and feel at peace with myself. I understand my past, which helps me to understand my needs today. My past was filled with physical and emotional pain, so I turned to pills to avoid further hurt. Dealing with my past head-on has allowed me to move toward a healthier future.*

> *I now feel worthy of a fulfilling life. I had always felt abandoned, both as a child and later as an adult. In therapy I worked through feelings of shame, loneliness and depression, so that I now have many healthy relationships.*

> *I learned to trust myself and others. Trust never came easy for me. I always thought that it was "a given," not an earned ability. I experienced rejection and told lies in the past. It wasn't until I began my recovery and went to support groups that I found trust, companionship and truth.*

> *I now feel I am a good person. Growing up, I was not shown a lot of support or affirmation. I didn't feel valued as a child. Through a very helpful network of people from support groups, I get affirmations, support and the feeling of being appreciated and valued.*

> *I have learned to take care of myself for the first time. I was so codependent with my family, I thought my purpose in life was to "fix" them; instead I lost myself. I have since worked diligently at taking care of myself through Al-Anon and other family support groups. I found out I can take care of myself while still being supportive of others, without "fixing" them.*

> *I have developed healthy ways of coping with stress and other uncomfortable feelings. Before recovery I would find unhealthy ways of dealing with emotional problems, such as overeating, undereating, drugs, gambling, sex, pills, anything to take the pain away. By sharing with other recovering people, I found healthier ways to relieve the pain I was feeling on the inside—a void that can only by talked out, not medicated.*

> *I have found balance in my life. I never felt any kind of balance in my life before. It was always in chaos; I was always living on the edge.*

> *I've learned to forgive myself. I felt guilty all the time about the hurt I must have inflicted upon family and friends. But most of all, I felt ashamed, never respecting or liking myself. I thought I was responsible for my disease. With help from therapy, support groups and my sponsor, I have learned that I am not responsible for my disease, but I am responsible for my recovery. Learning to forgive one's self doesn't come easy, but it does come.*

> *I deserve to be loved in a safe, nurturing environment. When I finally believed this statement was true, I knew I had made it.*

Here are some more thoughts about the joys of recovery from individuals who have shared their stories in this book. The first two are from the husbands of recovering prescription addicts.

My husband, Michael, speaks of family recovery:

I know we have been given a miraculous gift, for which I am very grateful. Our recovery is a lifelong journey, without ending, which means we will never be "cured." It means we have the tools to live a good life by recognizing the disease of addiction and what it is capable of and to take the steps necessary to keep it in check—as both the user and the codependent. It means altering our lifestyles to spend our lives together in a positive way and find happiness and contentment. The program really works, but it works a little bit differently for each person and it only works if you are willing to work for it! The longer we have been in recovery, the happier we have become. Our communication has blossomed to unimaginable heights as we both continue to remember and understand this disease that affects everyone in the family.

David, Shawna's husband, speaks of spiritual sustenance:

I am especially grateful to God for the miracle that He worked in my family's life. Without His help, I know there would have been no happy ending. I have discovered that God does not give up on any of us very easily. I almost hit the "panic button" with my wife and now I am so glad that I hung in there—even when things got really rough. God has miraculously restored the love and trust between my wife and me. Her recovery has brought our family back together, a feat I feared would never happen. "Healthy" is a word we thought only other families understood and felt. Now, we are healthy. We talk, we love and we play like we did when we dated. It's not to say things are perfect, but with each recovering day our lives together keep improving in some way. Our children have a mother again they can laugh with and talk to. A mother they can be proud of and a father who is full of pride. Together, we now carry God's message of hope and freedom to anyone who will listen.

Kevin speaks of self-growth:

I feel such gratitude for all the help I received through support groups, my sponsor and counselor. I have found new meaning and purpose in life. I've worked very hard to achieve self-respect and prove my worthiness to my family. In the beginning, I thought detoxification and treatment were all I needed to do to have a successful recovery. Others further along in the recovery process helped me understand that I needed to work on myself throughout my recovery program if I wanted to truly heal and keep what I now have—a life, a family and a career.

Pat speaks of insight:

I'm grateful to be alive today. I had to learn that I could survive on my own again without pills and without being a codependent of anyone. I needed to find help for dual illnesses in order to fight prescription addiction and severe depression. I needed more awareness of how I was raised and the understanding that my behavior was a result of a need to survive in an environment over which I had no control. Through recovery, I found the hope, understanding, guidance and structure I need to live a productive life. My ability to survive now comes from letting go of resentments and anger and empowering my own life, the way I choose to live it.

As for myself, I am now actually grateful for my disease, because the process of recovery has made such a positive impact on my life, giving me self-esteem, self-worth and a purpose in life. I think back and never want to forget who I was or where I came from. For it is my past that makes me who

I am today and what I will become tomorrow. I once thought I was unique and that my story and life were very different from everyone else's. I came to learn I wasn't so different or unique and that we are all in pursuit of personal growth and well-being. I have learned to freely share my pain, fear, anger and needs, never carrying the burden alone. I continue to ask for guidance from my "Higher Power" and try to live my life through the spiritual power of the Twelve Step principles. I will always be aware of this illness that I carry with me, never taking recovery for granted. My disease is what keeps me strong and motivated to keep improving myself. My journey continues to unfold as daily changes bring on new possibilities. My promise in recovery is to offer the help and wisdom that I have received and pass it on to others. I pray for the inner strength and courage to practice these principles in all that I do and say.

I am hoping to hear that you have made it, too.

EPILOGUE

When I got out of treatment and wanted to join a support group, I was directed to Alcoholics Anonymous and Narcotics Anonymous. The members of these groups are fine folks and I recommend their meetings. Some of their stories, however, were very different from mine and some of my needs were not met in their meetings. I missed being able to talk to someone about the aspects of recovery peculiar to prescription addiction. When I asked about support groups made up primarily of people with problems like mine, I found there were none. I was surprised, because I knew a bottle of pills was more likely to be found in a nearby purse or an unlocked medicine cabinet than a bottle of vodka or syringe full of heroin. It was those purses and cabinets I needed to guard against.

So I decided to form a group myself, inviting the people recovering from prescription addiction whom I'd met in the treatment center and in AA and NA. I called the new group Prescription Anonymous. Officials at the institution where I had been treated invited us to meet at that facility and we got off to a great start. When I was at Pennsylvania State University, I founded a group there for abused women and I was a facilitator for the group. Since then, I had been a healthcare educator, so I knew how to facilitate the new group. Prescription Anonymous has now grown and has chapters in other states.

When I had been clean a year, I chose to volunteer as a sponsor for two newly clean prescription addicts. I found this role very satisfying. The experience of helping others was rewarding to me and that focus also supported my own recovery.

When I began to write about my experience and those of others, I realized how even more widespread the problem of prescription addiction was than I had known. The blindsided feeling people expressed when they discovered they were addicted to a drug originally prescribed by a doctor made a huge impression on me. I thought there needed to be important changes made. At the same time, contact with recovering addicts in other states led me to take on a regional and national focus. I began to realize something had to be done about the dangers inherent in prescription drug abuse. I looked around, but little was being accomplished to stop this growing epidemic. Finally, I decided that I had to do something.

The next step was to find those who needed to become more aware and those who could help me bring attention to the problem.

The chart on the following page shows the groups and levels of responsibility which must ultimately be addressed if we are to end prescription and over-the-counter drug abuse.[1]

Opposite page: *Western Journal of Medicine*, 1990, Volume 152, page 614.
Reprinted with permission of BMJ Publishing Group and Donald R. Wesson.

PRESCRIPTION DRUG ABUSE AND RESPONSIBILITY

DRUG ENFORCEMENT
- To monitor sales
- To investigate diversion
- To enforce industry compliance with manufacturing quotas and sales

FOOD AND DRUG ADMINISTRATION
- To set production quotas of Schedule II controlled medications
- To review and approve package inserts
- To approve medications that are safe and efficacious

PHARMACEUTICAL MANUFACTURER
- To maintain manufacturing standards of purity and quality
- To avoid production in excess of quotas set by FDA
- To conform to industry standards in advertising and promotion of medications
- To report sales of controlled medications to DEA
- To provide information to physicians about the medications they manufacture
- To verify that customers who order medications from them are licensed to receive the medications

STATE PHARMACY LICENSING
- To license pharmacists who meet licensing requirements of the board
- To license and monitor pharmacies

STATE MEDICAL LICENSING BOARD
- To license physicians who meet the board's requirements
- To discipline mis-prescribing physicians

PHYSICIANS
- To examine and diagnose a patient's medical problems
- To prescribe appropriate medications based on a knowledge of the patient's conditions and history as well as other medications the patient may be taking
- To obtain current information about the medications they prescribe, including indications, side effects, therapeutic limitations and abuse potential

RETAIL PHARMACIES
- To dispense prescription medications prescribed by patients' physicians
- To follow regulations regarding dispensing of controlled medications
- To provide patient information about the medications

PATIENTS
- To be truthful with physicians
- To follow physicians' instructions
- To take medications as prescribed

PATIENTS

As you can see from the responsibilities of patients listed at the bottom of the chart, the patient is the first one who must be made accountable for proper use of medication. The American Medical Association states that while healthcare providers who fail in their responsibilities to patients should be censured, the current tendencies to assign fault to physicians when patients have violated their responsibility is unreasonable and unfair to physicians. When patients are dishonest in the patient-physician relationship and deceive their doctors or when patients use their medications other than as prescribed, society should hold the patients, not physicians, accountable for the inevitable adverse consequences. Because the patient is responsible for herself, my primary goal is to first educate the patient so that she can make responsible choices.

PHYSICIANS

Next on the hierarchy of those responsible are physicians. If physicians, including dentists, prescribed wisely and knew their patients' histories and other medications the patients were taking, the chances for prescription addiction to occur would be reduced. Moreover, requests for prescription refills of pain medications, sleeping pills, etc., should raise red flags for all doctors. Doctors should consider patients' histories and current medical conditions and re-evaluate patients who ask for refills, so that they are aware of any changes. In the case of children, like Shawna, who became addicted through the use of prescribed painkillers at an early age, certainly children have no responsibility for use or misuse. Though well meaning, doctors must be vigilant when prescribing powerful and addictive drugs to children, particularly those who are not old enough to understand the consequences of addiction. In such cases, doctors should inform parents about the possibility of addiction, the warning signs and how and where to get help. When treating adults, doctors must apprise them of all potential side effects—including addiction. These newly-educated, responsible patients, in concert with well-trained, responsible doctors, will be equipped to avoid addiction.

The following guide is an elaboration of the responsibilities of physicians and patients.

RESPONSIBILITIES OF PHYSICIANS AND PATIENTS
IN THE PHYSICIAN-PATIENT INTERACTION

Physician

To have the patient's well-being as his or her primary concern

To formulate a working diagnosis of the patient's problem based on the patient's history and examination

To obtain the appropriate laboratory test or consultation with a specialist to clarify diagnosis

To prescribe appropriate therapy (assumes that the physician is acting within his or her scope of expertise and that the physician possesses about the same level of knowledge as other practitioners in the community)

To monitor the effect of treatment, including monitoring for side effects of toxicity

To continue follow-up until the condition is resolved or the patient's care is assumed by another physician

Patient

To seek medical attention for conditions that he or she believes a physician can cure or ameliorate

To be truthful in relating historical information and to cooperate with the physical examination

To cooperate in obtaining the laboratory tests—or consultations—requested by the physician

To comply with the physician's instructions, such as taking medications as prescribed and avoiding activities that would complicate or aggravate the disease

To report symptoms accurately

To follow through with follow-up appointments until discharged by the physician

It is the responsibility of the physician to prescribe the least addictive medication possible for as short a time as the patient needs and only as necessary. It is also the physician's responsibility to warn patients if prescribed medications are addictive. Of course, some prescriptions of careful and honest physicians indicate a limited number of refills without reevaluation. However, unlimited refills can be dangerous. Physicians expect their patients to follow instructions. Many physicians think that the insert enclosed in the packaging of the medication suffices, but that is an unwise assumption to make. Few patients read the inserts to learn the degree of addictiveness—their most immediate concern is relief of their symptoms. Doctors must simply take the time to tell patients when medications are both effective and addictive. For every addictive medication prescribed, the doctor should say, "I don't want you to suffer in pain, but I don't want you to get dependent on these pills either. Take no more than you need and try to stop using them as soon as possible. There is no reason to finish the bottle." When it comes to medications like antibiotics, patients are used to being told to take all the pills in the bottle even if they feel better. Thus, it is important to emphasize the fact that it is not necessary to do the same when taking addictive medications like painkillers.

In addition, all physicians and dentists should be aware of the patterns of deceit addicted patients use to get pills. Here are some requests the addicted patient might make that should send up red flags.

Patient to Doctor:
> I'm going on vacation for two to three weeks (the second or third time this patient has had a similar request over the last several months); can I have enough pills to last me until I get back?

> I'm having pain and can't sleep at night! I heard you were the best in your field (flattery). I can't find anyone that seems to be able to help me with my pain and your name was given to me by one of your patients. (The name will be a made-up one, but doctors don't remember the names of all their patients anyway.)

> I have migraines daily; I need a stronger pill!

> A family member just died and I can't sleep.

> My husband and I are having problems; my anxiety is out of control.

Patient to Nurses or Staff:
> Can I get another refill on my prescription? Dr. _____ said I could call **you** if I was still having pain or I couldn't sleep. Here's my pharmacy

number and Rx refill number so it will be <u>easy for you</u> to call it in for me. (It sounds like the patient is doing the nurse a favor.)

Patient to Emergency Room Staff:
>   I couldn't get an appointment with my doctor and couldn't stand the pain any longer.

Patient to Intern or Physician's Assistant:
>   Same scenario as physician listed above, but Physician Assistants and interns are sometimes easier to persuade, because they are so eager to help the suffering that they believe the addict and forget to ask probing questions that may put up a red-flag.

Patient to Doctor on call:
>   My personal doctor is not available this weekend and I was hoping you could give me a refill. I have an appointment set up later this month with my regular doctor. Can I have enough pills to last until my appointment?

Patient to Dentist:
>   The tooth that you worked on last week still hurts and the pills you gave me don't seem to be strong enough.
>   I have another toothache that is bothering me; perhaps that's the one with a cavity and it needs pulling. Can you give me something for pain until I can get in to your office?

Healthcare workers hear all these requests and more. But it is important for them to consider that such requests may be the ploys of addicts. Here are some other suggestions to help doctors avoid feeding patients' habits.

>   If you suspect that a patient may be drug seeking, don't leave a patient alone in the exam room. Ask a nurse or assistant to stay in the room with the patient while you leave for a minute. If there is no one available at the time, leave the exam door open a little. This may discourage a patient from opening drawers and cabinets.
>   Never leave your prescription pad in the exam room, on the counter or in a drawer, while a patient is unattended or at the nurses' station where someone can pick it up.
>   Don't ever place expired pills in an open trash basket.
>   Always document on patient charts the instructions verbally given

and copy all written prescriptions as well as instructions for sample medications handed out.

> Use prescription pads with patterns that make alteration difficult and triplicate copy forms for protection against forgery.

> Write out in words as well as numerals the number of pills you're dispensing so that your patient can't add any extra numbers to the written prescription.

> Except in cases of real emergencies, healthcare providers or dentists should not call in new or refill prescriptions over the phone.

> Be observant while talking to your patients. Do her eyes look watery or red? Look for unusual nervousness. Can he sit still? Does your patient look at you while you're talking? Is he interested in your diagnosis or just interested in getting a prescription and getting out of there? Is her overall demeanor unusually sluggish and does she look disconnected from reality? Does he look and act depressed? All of these could be signs of substance abuse.

> Read previous office notes about each patient and look at medications written in the past, including the number of refills allowed. A red flag should go up if you see that an unusual or unjustified amount of pills have been prescribed without sufficient need.

> Communication with all staff members who have contact with patients should include reporting any suspicious activity and developing a plan of action should anyone suspect a patient is drug seeking.

> Most state laws indicate that any healthcare provider can discharge a patient with written and verbal notice with "just cause" if the provider believes that a patient has come to them under false pretense or if there is proof of fraud or forgery. Call the referring physicians, pharmacists or dentists and ask if they have ever questioned or had problems with the patient's attempts to obtain prescriptions. Ask how many addictive prescriptions the patient has been given in the past three, six and twelve months and how many refills and in what time frame.

> Remember that healthcare providers not only have an obligation to help their patients avoid addiction, but they must also protect the clinic or hospital they work for against liability for wrongdoing.

> When dismissing any patient who you suspect has an addiction to pills or other drugs, use gentleness and compassion along with firmness in your explanation. Some patients may have started coming to you with real pain and suffering only to have gotten addicted to the very substance you prescribed. Confront your patient in your office (with a witness), showing

your proof or reason for suspicion. Let him know you are obligated to dismiss him, but then offer names and places where he might go for help.

PHARMACISTS

Pharmacists are an important link in the chain of addiction. Customers con pharmacists as often as physicians. Here are some good policies for pharmacists and pharmacy personnel to adopt:

> Do not allow anyone to pick up a prescription at a pharmacy without showing identification first, especially at the drive-through service.

> To avoid theft, do not leave filled prescriptions within reach of customers. In fact, do not leave prescriptions within reading distance as information for deceit is sometimes gleaned by sharp-eyed addicts who read labels of other people's bottles and claim to be that person.

> Shred all prescriptions and records of prescriptions before discarding to prevent addicts from getting old prescriptions or information such as DEA numbers from the trash.

> Pharmacists should always review medications to clarify use and addictive capabilities and make sure the patient looks at the warnings indicated on the bottle, enclosed with the packaging or distributed by the pharmacy.

> Pharmacists should document any suspicions of abuse or fraudulent activities and notify the healthcare provider and law enforcement.

> Pharmacists should be wary of requests like these: "It's the weekend and my doctor's office is closed, can I have just a few pills until Monday or until he gets back from vacation?" or "I put some of these in a travel case and I lost it. Can you give me just a few pills to make up for the ones I lost?"

Like all healthcare providers, pharmacists should confront patients who they suspect of drug abuse when choosing not to fill their prescriptions. Again, gentleness and compassion along with information on treatment options may make a difference. It's true, most addicts will go to another pharmacy, but by refusing to fill some prescription you may help a drug abuser to seek help. Consider this letter I received:

I turned in a prescription from a different doctor to my pharmacist. He caught it immediately. He pulled me over to the side of the counter and told me how dangerous and addictive these drugs were. He told me how easy it was to get addicted and that it happens to a lot of people. He suggested that

I was an addict. That made me mad. I didn't like what he said, because he exposed my problem. I knew he knew and I wasn't ready to own up to the addiction. He made it very hard on me to cheat. If one thing was wrong with the prescription, he wouldn't fill it. He really cared. When I straightened up, I realized what a great man he was. After I recovered, I told him everything—I even printed out my story from the drug abuse site and gave it to him. He had already looked it up—I just didn't know it. I consider him a dear friend.

While there is no evidence that the pharmacist was responsible for this addict's recovery, his diligence was probably one of the important factors that pushed her to admit she had a problem and seek help.

LICENSING BOARDS

You should report to the state medical licensing board any doctor who blatantly contributes to addiction by overprescribing or prescribing without sufficient oversight or while ignoring clear signs of patient abuse. Drug abuse by physicians themselves should also be reported. Retain all evidence of misconduct. While many physicians retain their licenses even with clear evidence of their failing their responsibilities and even after convictions for drug misuse, your complaint will be registered and will be on that doctor's record for public scrutiny. Your complaint may contribute to the physician curtailing the abuse.

Likewise report to the pharmacy board any pharmacist who dispenses addictive medications without prescription or honors an obviously falsified prescription.

These measures are intended to help prevent prescription addiction or prevent addicts from easily getting inappropriate prescriptions filled. The harder it is to continue addictive behavior, the more likely the addict is to turn to treatment for relief. The goal is to make it easier to get treatment than to get the drugs to feed the addiction.

Just as I have found great satisfaction and, hopefully, have made a difference by spreading the word about prescription addiction, so you can help by being aware of the problem, understanding that addiction is an illness, telling all who will listen that treatment is available and recovery is possible and worth the effort. To all those who are fighting to recover, I send my heartfelt encouragement. To those of you who are recovering, I send congratulations. I hope you will reach out to other addicts who need your guidance and understanding in order to take the first step to recovery.

PRESCRIPTION:
FOR ALL DOCTORS AND PRESCRIPTION ADDICTS

Healthy Choices – Make them and live by them!
Directions: Use every day
Refills: A lifetime

Individuals recovering from chemical or substance abuse, <u>do</u> <u>not</u> use caution while on this prescription. Reported side effects: Happiness, growth and serenity.

- Signed and approved by all who have listened and learned

APPENDIX 1:

Questions and Answers

Over the years, recovering prescription addicts have asked me many questions. Most of the answers can be found in this book, but I've found that people often don't absorb general information directly into their own context; they need to ask about their individual situations. The following is a question and answer section which I hope will address some of your concerns.

First, here are some questions frequently asked by family members and loved ones.

Concerns of Friends and Families of Prescription Addicts

Q: I've been married to this person for years; I should have known there was something wrong, shouldn't I have?

A: No. Some addicts can be the best actors in the world. Despite the perfect vision of hindsight, if you are not aware of the dangers or the signs, it is easy to miss addiction. Just as you wouldn't see a disease like cancer coming, neither would you see the disease of addiction. Don't feel guilty about not knowing. However, do learn all you can about addiction now.

Q: I have a friend I believe is hooked on pills. We are close, but she has never told me about any problem with drugs. Suppose one day she tells me about her addiction and voluntarily asks me for help. Does this ever happen? Of course, I'd say yes, but what should I say next?

A: When someone says, "I need help," ask, "Do you really want help?" This question jolts the person. It also makes her say, "Yes, I need help" again as an affirmation of commitment. Then respond, "Let's go to a doctor." Immediately find a doctor, make an appointment and take your friend there yourself. Constantly reassure her that things will work out and you will be there by her side when she needs you.

Q: My family wants to do an intervention as soon as possible with our addicted father. What are the chances we can do it without an intervention professional?

A: Addiction, as I have said many times, is a family disease. The behavior of family members has revolved around the addiction even, to some extent, if they have not known about the addiction until recently. The intervention will shake up everyone's life, not just the addict's. Preparation for an intervention with a professional might act as the first session of therapy for the family. That would definitely be a positive thing. Everyone would be starting with the same information and the same strategy.

The danger of going into intervention without professional counseling is that some family problems could come out during the intervention that would distract everyone from the main purpose. The result would be a breakdown in the family's united front. For example, if a family member who went along with the plan suddenly blurted out that he didn't think the problem was that bad anyway, an argument might ensue, letting the addict off the hook. Or, if one family member blamed another for the problem, someone else might defend the accused person and suddenly everyone is taking sides. Such a situation would not help the addicted person at all and would only make matters worse for him or her and the entire family. A trained professional experienced in intervention could handle the discord and lead you all to more productive behavior.

If you must do an intervention without help, practice what each person is going to say ahead of time and find out what the feelings of each person are so that problematic issues have been brought out in the open and dealt with ahead of time. You may get a feeling during practice about whether these people are going to work together well or not. Furthermore, if you feel you "have to" do the intervention without professional help, that suggests you are trying to keep the whole matter hidden. Such a need for secrecy doesn't speak well for the overall healthy approach to a problem whose solution requires honesty. Addiction is a disease, so get professional help.

Q: Our daughter is addicted to pills. We have sent her to therapy and even had her in treatment once. We've given her money, support, housing, food and clothes—at this point what else can we do?

A: At some point you have to get on with your life, too. This disease will take the family down with it if you allow it. If you have done all you can do without destroying the rest of the family, tell your daughter that you will always love her, but that you can't let her live with you and you can't give her money, clothes, etc. anymore. Tell her you hope she will recover and you will be happy when that happens. Withdrawing support may even jolt her into getting serious about recovery. In the meantime, you may need therapy to help you with this tough love approach. You do have to take care of yourself, too, just as the addict has to take care of herself.

Those who stand on the sidelines and wish they could do something to save their friend, partner or family member from self-destruction eventually realize that no matter how many good intentions, wishes and earnest efforts they have for a loved one, ultimately it's entirely and exclusively up to the addicted person. As one family member said to me, "You can't will someone to live any more than you can will someone to die."

Q: I think we will be able to get our son taken to a hospital for treatment when he is very sick, but you say the addict has to want to recover. Our son doesn't seem to want to recover as much as we want him to. So will forcing him into treatment work or will it just be a waste of our money?

A: It is true that someone who is forced to face his addiction by the police, his family or his friends may not really be facing it; instead, he goes through treatment to please others, not because he is really committed to change. He will have trouble complying with treatment and have difficulty opening up, because he can't open his mind to the possibilities that he has an illness. For him, there is a high risk of relapse and less likelihood that he will stay in treatment. Even so, treatment to which a person is not open at first may open a door that has previously been closed. Plenty of people have sincerely faced their illness after detoxing in a treatment center; they have accepted help and gone on to recover. No one can say if your son will open his heart to recovery and take responsibility or not. The only sure thing is that he will probably never recover if he does not go to a treatment center, so in that sense, it's worth the risk.

Q: Our bills are never paid on time. Important appointments are never kept. Promises to our children are always broken. Pills have become a more important part of my husband's life than his family. There's no sign of this changing. I don't want to endure everything you have to go through to get a person to recover. I want to leave. What do you say to someone like me who just isn't willing to stick it out?

A: Only you can decide what you are willing to go through to assist the recovery of a loved one. If you have something between you that you feel is worth saving, get therapy for yourself, enlist the help of a professional, try an intervention. Make your decision to leave part of the intervention. You can say to your husband that you will leave if he doesn't get treatment. Or, if you are not willing to see it through, you can say that you are leaving anyway and you hope he gets treatment. Either way, you have given your husband a shot at sobriety. You have let him know that life cannot go on as before. It is your decision. I recommend therapy for you and your children no matter what happens.

Q: My mother died of prescription addiction. Our family is left with so many "what ifs," "if onlys" and "should haves" that we wish could have been answered before it was too late.

A: I am sorry about your great loss. Maybe you could have done something differently and it would have saved your mother's life, but maybe not. Recovery is up to the individual. You cannot make someone recover even if you do all the right things. We all wish we had done some things differently in life. If you are consumed with guilt, please get therapy for yourself and the family. If you want a way to "do something" about it now, help publicize the dangers of misusing prescription drugs, work to get legislation in your state changed and be available to talk to families about what you now know.

Concerns of People in Recovery

Q: I admit that I am powerless over my addiction and I cannot control my behavior. I just cannot face admitting this to my family, so I am putting off getting help. How can I get the courage to tell them?

A: Many families are relieved to hear an announcement such as yours, because they already knew or had some idea. There's a good chance they will be very supportive. However, I understand your fear. Ironically, your family is probably also dealing with a lot of their own fears. They may fear you are going to blame them. They may exclaim, "How could you!" Or they might minimize your addiction, complaining that they can't understand why you can't simply read the instructions on the bottle and take your medicine as directed. They may say you can recover on your own; you don't need psychiatrists and treatment centers. What they are really telling you when they say these things is that they are afraid, too. If you go into treatment, your addiction will be out in the open and they may fear shame and embarrassment. Furthermore, they may have adapted to your disease, whether in a healthy manner or not. They have developed a routine. When you change, they must change. Some family members are very frightened of what your change is going to mean for them, even though they will say they want you to stop abusing your prescriptions. They may have been enabling you in your helplessness; now they are going to have to support you in a different, yet equally difficult venture. Their roles will change. They may not be ready.

Knowing family members may be acting out of fear as great as yours may help you face their reactions. Explain to them that you need to make this change and that you must put your struggle first—even before them. Tell them you may need to maintain some distance from your family and friends for a time. Ask for their support without judgment or criticism. To their accusing "How could you?" simply say, "I have to learn about my addiction first before I can explain it to you." Once you have decided to put recovery first, you cannot worry about them. Be self-centered. In the end, those around you will benefit from your recovery. And in the end, you can reconnect with loved ones. You will be able to explain addiction and recovery to them or, if you prefer, you can just show them what a wonderful thing recovery is by your behavior and newfound joy in life without addiction.

Q: How can I get in touch with Prescription Anonymous?

A: The phone number for this organization is 770-428-1220 and the Web site is www.prescriptionanonymous.org.

Q: I have been through detox and feel that I need help. I haven't prayed very much in my life. I don't know how to start. Is there a prayer you could give me that would work?

A: Prayer doesn't "work" unless you work. God helps those who help themselves. A prayer certainly can get you in the right frame of mind to do what you have to do. The following is a well-known prayer that was adapted for prescription addicts.

God, grant me the Courage to admit that I am powerless over my addiction to any mood altering substance and co-occurring illnesses, the Wisdom that I gain through support groups, sponsors, and prayer, so that I may share with others

*who still suffer, and the Serenity that comes from within, which
can be felt not only by me, but those I choose to have in my life.*

Q: How do I find doctors and other people who understand my disease?"

A: Get recommendations from other recovering addicts you meet in treatment and support groups. Also check my Web site and the resources listed in appendix II.

Q: How do I keep from going back into denial?

A: Here are some things you can do to stay honest with yourself:

Keep a journal in which you record feelings, moods and anger-provoking situations as they arise. Include the intensity of your feelings and how you dealt with them. This record helps you track your mood changes over time so that you can learn from them and share your findings with your sponsor or therapist.

Talk about your guilt and shame. Addicts often feel extremely guilty and shameful about a disease over which they have no control. They may feel guilty over things said in anger to their families, spouses, children, even co-workers, when they were really angry at themselves. In recovery, they may feel guilty about not paying more attention to others instead of focusing all their energy on themselves. They are ashamed of their failings. If you are experiencing these feelings, discuss them in treatment and at support group meetings. The understanding you receive in group meetings gives you the support you need to deal with these issues.

Learn to forgive yourself. For most addicts this is one of the toughest steps to take. You are not responsible for your disease, but you are responsible for your recovery. You can't forget your past and may not be able to make amends to all those you have harmed, but you do have control over your future. If you're doing all the right things to change your behavior, you will become healthier and happier and, if you keep recovery first in your life, time will heal you and you will be able to forgive yourself.

Identify feelings of loss. Some people have a strong sense of loss or grief after stopping their abuse of pills. They become depressed and withdrawn as if they lost a loved one or a job. In a sense you really have lost something that was once close to you, something that gave you a sense of security. Share your feelings of loss and depression with your therapist or in group support meetings. Soon, a healthier life and positive behaviors will be more fulfilling than pills and will replace your loss.

Q: I had some friends before I got clean who used drugs and drank. I still like them and I wish they were in recovery, too. I hate to cut them off when they call me. Do you have to give up your friends? That makes recovery hard and sad.

A: Friends are indeed valuable. You need friends more now than ever before. However, most people in recovery cannot keep the same friends they had when they were abusing drugs, because those friends may have been as ill as the addicts were. Remember, changing old behaviors isn't easy. If you go back to your old friends, you will be tempted to go back to your old ways. Staying in recovery comes first, always, above all else.

Yes, you will need friends. New friends. You need the healing powers of a good friend, someone you feel comfortable with, someone who will listen without judgment or criticism. You need someone who won't lie to you, but, more importantly, who won't allow you to lie to him. Friendships keep you planted solidly on the ground and help you to feel peace. Choosing a friend is very important, especially in recovery. Choose wisely someone who will be a benefit to you, someone who does not abuse or misuse prescription medications or mind altering substances. Many of us meet these new friends in support groups.

Tell the old friends who call and who still use mind-altering substances that it is very important to you to recover and that you must be away from them for a while. Tell them you hope they, too, will get treatment and that you will do all you can to encourage them when that time comes. Maybe your recovery will inspire them to follow suit. That is surely the best way for you to show your friendship. But for now, stay away.

Q: Is there some easy way to know when I am in danger of relapse? I seem to get too down in the dumps before I realize what's happening. I need to recognize danger sooner.

A: In chapter 8 there are lists of situations which will help you recognize the triggers for relapse. I suggest you read over the list every week or so to help you recognize what's happening in your life. Also, one therapist taught a recovering addict this acronym: H.A.L.T. It means: hurt, angry, lonely, tired. These states will trigger compulsive actions. When you feel hurt, angry, lonely or tired, change your behavior and surroundings. Do something soothing, call a friend or sponsor and get some rest.

Q: I thought if I took one or two extra pills for my stress that I would feel better faster and I wouldn't have to think about my problems. That ruined my life. I've finally given up the pills and now my problems seem worse than ever. What can I do besides start taking pills again?

A: You will have to treat both the addiction and the original problem that you were trying to mask through pills. At least half of all prescription addicts have a dual diagnosis of addiction and depression or some other psychological problem. Find a therapist who understands both addiction and other psychological disorders. Join a recovery group where you will find peers who understand.

Q: On top of all the other painful emotions I had before, I now have the shame of knowing how badly I hurt the people I care about while I was on prescription drugs. That's just one more thing to worry about in recovery. How can I face the people I've hurt?

A: You've already hurt these people and your relationships can't really get worse. The only thing they can do is improve. Think through what you honestly feel now that you have taken responsibility for your behavior. Rehearse your speech and prepare to listen to their responses without defensiveness. Your therapist can help you plan your approach. Tell them that you now realize and regret how much you have hurt them. Speak calmly, no matter what. Almost always the hurt person's response is better than you expected. It almost always helps your relationship enormously. Moreover, when you take responsibility for what you did, the other person often volunteers that he sees he had a part in the original problem, too. In any case, both of you will feel better when you reach out honestly and contritely to those you have hurt. You will probably find they are on your side more than ever before.

Q: I am sober and supposedly in recovery. I still feel like killing myself sometimes. I think I'll never make it. Is it really worth the struggle?

A: Yes. You are probably depressed and you never learned the normal skills for facing the problems in life because you relied on pills to relieve stress. Talk to a psychiatrist who can help you with not only the addiction, but your emotional problems as well. Or, see another kind of therapist plus an addictionologist or physician knowledgeable about addiction and addictive medications.

Q: I was diagnosed with addiction and depression. How can my doctor take away my pills without making my depression worse?

A: You are right that doing without your pills may leave you depressed. You are also right that depression may require medication similar to the pills to which you were addicted. The new treatment will be using non-addictive drugs at much lower doses, which will be effective now that you are detoxed. Your physician must be one who understands addiction and you must tell every doctor, dentist and pharmacist you ever see for any kind of problem that you are an addict so that he or she can keep you on a low risk regimen of medication.

Q: Can over-the-counter medications be addictive? Which ones can I take that would be low risk?

A: Yes, over-the-counter medications can be addictive if they are abused, that is, if you take more than directed. Some contain addictive components similar to what is in prescription medication, just in lower doses. Refer to page 123 in chapter 8 for a list of over-the-counter medications considered low risk by a pharmacist.

Q: I can't talk to my family or friends; they don't believe I have a disease called *prescription addiction*. How can I make them understand?

A: It's pretty hard for you to stop abusing drugs, learn new skills, change your lifestyle and at the same time educate your family and convince disbelieving relatives that the problem you have is not just sleazy behavior. Don't try. Tell the family once, repeat it once more if necessary and then let them be. To overcome addiction, you have to concentrate on you and your life. You have to let what others say slide and leave convincing them for another day. This is a time when others who know about prescription addiction from experience should become your confidants and friends. This is one reason support groups are so important.

Q: My husband and I are having difficulty talking to each other about my disease. He doesn't trust me. How do we go on from here?

A: Of course he doesn't trust you. You've probably lied to him a hundred times to hide your addiction and emotions. Now, you must say what you need to say, being open and truthful—and brave—and then don't worry about what he says back. Don't try to talk him into trust. Concentrate on you. In time, your changed behavior will convince him that you are becoming worthy of his trust again.

Q: I am truly sorry for how I have hurt my family and I want to make amends. I am terrified and don't know what to say.

A: Start with the short statement, "I am very sorry for how I have hurt you." Just that simple apology is a release and sometimes is enough to reestablish comfort and repair broken bonds. As an example, consider what I told my father when I tried to make amends. I had hurt his feelings. I had stopped showing respect and wasn't talking to him. When I finally found the courage to try to repair our relationship, I said, "I am really sorry I have hurt you." I also said that he had hurt me and I had to deal with that. He said, "I do feel badly that I didn't handle things as well as I should have." That made me feel that I didn't bear the whole burden of our estrangement and reconciliation. We were both sorry and we wanted to reconnect. My father and I are close now and he is proud of my recovery and how I help other people.

Q: My husband and I are planning our first trip since I have been in recovery. I am worried that since our routine will be different for a few days, I won't be able to handle it. There will be tensions and temptations. Is there anything I can do to make this trip safer for me?

A: As with any successful vacation or trip, planning ahead is essential. You will likely plan your itinerary, activities and visits with friends and family. Why not include planning ahead for scheduled support meetings to attend as well? Look in the white or yellow pages of any telephone book for Prescription Anonymous, Dual Recovery Anonymous, Alcoholics Anonymous or Narcotics Anonymous. Call and ask about the locations closest to where you will be vacationing. Get the days and times and plan on attending as many meetings as you need to. I promise you that people in support groups anywhere you go will be just as receptive, kind and welcoming as your own support group at home. Many people don't realize that even cruise ships have twelve-step recovery support meetings. The meetings will be listed as "Friends of Bill W." on the cruise schedule of activities, a code word that protects your privacy from those less in the know.

Also, before your trip, try to make arrangements to have a car available to you at all times so you are not on anyone else's schedule but your own. This way, if you are feeling anxious or stressed, you can go for a quiet drive to gather your thoughts. You can certainly call your sponsor long distance just as readily as when you are at home.

Q: How do I act when I go back to work? What do I say about my absence?

A: If no one at work knows of your addiction, you have options. You could simply state that you got into trouble with prescription drugs and you had to take some time to recover. That would help spread a warning to others about the dangers of abusing prescription drugs. If you think it would be to your advantage to keep your addiction private or if you just choose to do so, tell people you have had a health problem, give few details and stick to this account. To any additional questions, say, "I'm trying to put my illness behind me and I'd feel better if I didn't talk about it." Your behavior and skills at work, no longer subject to the effects of inappropriate drugs, will build your colleagues' trust in your competence. If, on the other hand, some people know about your addiction, you can still tell them whatever truth you want about the problem or you can still say, "I'm trying to put my illness behind me now that I have recovered, so I'd prefer to not talk about it." Additionally, if your work was stressful before treatment and recovery, seriously consider seeking a new job that would make you happier. A better job might have more routine or more variety, more action or a slower pace, whatever will not tempt you to medicate for stress. It is better to earn less and be at peace than to earn more and never know when you will feel the desire to take a mind-altering substance to help you "get through a crisis."

Q: I have been in recovery for a year and therefore I'm eligible to be a sponsor. I don't know if I am ready for this or if I even want to do it. What are the pros and cons of agreeing to sponsor others?

A: People who have been in recovery for a year or more often find they enjoy becoming sponsors and facilitators at support groups. They also feel sponsorship helps them continue their recovery more easily. The following comments of sponsors I know address this question: "Newcomers remind me where I was and being a sponsor reinforces my own recovery." "It keeps me tuned-in and aware of my own problems as well as my own progress." "Listening to newcomers reminds me I can be right back to where they are at any time. No one is immune to relapse." As you teach newly sober people, you are reinforcing the lessons you need to remember forever yourself. Helping people also gives you a good feeling and helps your own self-esteem. I personally have as strong an urge to help someone now as I used to have to find help. If you don't have this desire, perhaps you are not ready to take the step of sponsorship. Don't feel guilty about it; sponsorship is not for everyone.

Q: I am in recovery and I know I must remember that I am still an addict so I won't relapse. But I'm so tired of my life revolving around being an addict and always thinking about codependence and enabling and trying not to be part of a dysfunctional family. Is there ever any other way of looking at it?

A: I agree that so much attention must be given to the dysfunction of the family and so much is said about the disease that you forget you can eventually be a part of a healthy family. Someday you will get beyond these troubled times. Then you will need to change your mind-set. You will no longer have a dysfunctional family but a "functional" family. To encourage "another way of looking at it," Prescription Anonymous members came up with the following acronym with its positive elaboration. Perhaps this acronym will help you look at the brighter side:

FUNCTIONAL

F: Freedom of expression: Each of us holds the power and right to perceive, to want and desire, to exhibit emotion, to make choices and to change.

U: Uninterrupted attention given to each other: Couples need to set aside time to listen to each other without interruption.

N: Negotiated differences: To negotiate differences there must first be the desire to cooperate and a willingness to hear other viewpoints and concerns.

C: Communication: Clear communication requires respect for one's self and others as well as effort and skill.

T: Trust. Trust is created by honesty. Express yourself honestly. Sharing emotion, thoughts and fears is more important then agreement.

I: Individuality: Individual differences between members of the family should be encouraged. Families often learn from one another. Our own uniqueness should be honored.

O: Open-mindedness: Family members should be open-minded and flexible with each other so that each person can be spontaneous without fear, guilt or shame.

N: Needs fulfilled: Couples and families that get their needs met feel respected, loved, important and happy. Express your needs and your appreciation when they are met.

A: Accountability: You each (through treatment or therapy) know what your part in recovery is. Be responsible for your part and acknowledge when you have made mistakes.

L: Love: Love is allowing loved ones to make mistakes and find solutions for themselves. Love is patient, kind and forgiving.

This last question is the one I'm asked most often. I hope my answer will reassure you.

Q: Will I ever be happy again?

A: Yes, when you have overcome prescription addiction, you will be happier than you ever were before. I am living proof—and I have many new friends who are living proof. Sobriety opens a new world of possibilities and accomplishments. The process of recovery helps you grow, have confidence in yourself, set goals, learn new skills and relate to people in a healthier way. Recovery allows you to find your purpose and move on with your life holding your head high. I'm pulling for you.

APPENDIX 2:
Resources

This section contains a list of resources for addicts and their loved ones. Included are support groups, national government agencies and state addiction prevention programs. These groups and organizations can provide answers to questions or direct you to other appropriate sources.

SUPPORT GROUPS

Prescription Anonymous (RxA)
P.O. Box 1297
Powder Springs, GA 30127-1297
(770) 428-1220

Prescription Anonymous is a twelve-step program offering hope to the millions of people who are afflicted with addiction to prescription and over-the-counter medications and co-occurring illnesses. Together, members learn how to cope, change and make responsible choices.

Dual Recovery Anonymous (DRA)
1302 Division Street, Suite 101
Nashville, TN 37203
(615) 742-1000
(888) 869-9230

Dual Recovery Anonymous (DRA) is a self-help program based on the principles of the twelve steps, experiences of people in dual recovery and the principles of freedom and choice that are related to both chemical dependency and emotional or psychiatric illness.

Benzodiazepine Anonymous (BA)
6333 Wilshire Blvd., Suite 506
Los Angeles, CA 90048
(310) 652-4100

A twelve-step support group that helps people live free from physical and psychological dependence on benzodiazepines/sedatives such as Xanax, Librium, Ativan, Valium and Halcion. Members share their own stories, offering support and understanding through their experiences.

Narcotics Anonymous (NA)
P.O. Box 9999
Van Nuys, CA 91409
(818) 773-9999

Members learn to live drug free through the twelve-steps and twelve traditions adapted from Alcoholics Anonymous World Services. They focus on all addictions rather than specific or co-occurring illnesses. NA is a non-profit, international, community-based organization.

Alcoholics Anonymous (AA)
P.O. Box 459
Grand Central Station
New York, NY 10163
(212) 870-3400

Alcoholics Anonymous, a twelve-step recovery program, is a fellowship of women and men who share with each other their experiences, strengths and hopes to help in recovery from alcoholism. The focus is primarily on alcohol recovery and families of alcoholics.

Al-Anon Family Groups
1600 Corporate Landing Parkway
Virginia Beach, VA 23454-5617
(757) 563-1600

Al-Anon is worldwide organization that offers a program of recovery for the families and friends of alcoholics and other addictions whether or not the loved one seeks help. Members offer comfort and understanding that binds individuals and groups together through mutual exchanges of experiences, strengths and hopes.

INFORMATIONAL AGENCIES

Foundations Associates
1302 Division Street, Suite 101
Nashville, TN 37203
(615) 742-1000
(888) 869-9230

Foundations Associates (affiliated with Dual Recovery Anonymous) specializes in the treatment of individuals with a dual diagnosis, affected by both an emotional or psychiatric illness and chemical dependency. Foundations Associates provides a sober transition into the community by offering comprehensive, client-centered treatment, supportive housing and educational services to assist dual-diagnosed individuals and their families.

American Pharmaceutical Association
2215 Constitution Avenue, NW
Washington, DC 20037-2985
(202) 628-4410
(800) 237-2742

APHA Foundation distributes health information to the general public and offers continuing education programs for pharmacists. APHA is a professional organization of pharmacists and specialists who understand the correct use of medicines. Pharmacists dispense drugs according to healthcare providers and can answer questions about non-prescription products sold in pharmacies.

American Psychiatric Association
1400 K Street, NW
Washington, DC 20005
(202) 682-6239
Fax (202) 682-6850

APA is a professional society of psychiatrists and medical doctors who specialize in treating individuals with mental or emotional disorders. The association continues to research and improve the diagnosis, treatment and rehabilitation of individuals through continued education programs for psychiatrists. Individuals can contact the Association to locate a psychiatrist in their area for consultation.

Center for Substance Abuse Prevention (CSAP)
5600 Fishers Lane
Rockville, MD 20857
(301) 443-0373
(800) 729-6686

CSAP provides national leadership in the federal effort to prevent the use of alcohol, tobacco and other drugs which have been linked to serious national problems: rising health costs, crime, violence, school failure, HIV/AIDS, teen pregnancy and low work productivity. CSAP produces an array of informational and educational tools including telephone helplines.

National Institute on Drug Abuse (NIDA)
P.O. Box 30652
Bethesda, MD 20824-0652
(301) 443-1677
(888) 644-6432

NIDA is a federal government agency developing effective strategies to deal with problems and issues associated with alcohol and drug abuse. They provide information to healthcare professionals and the public on the risks and consequences of drug and alcohol abuse. Researchers funded by the Institute work to identify new ways to prevent substance abuse.

STATE PROGRAMS FOR ADDICTION PREVENTION

Alabama
Substance Abuse Division
100 N. Union Street
Montgomery, AL 36130
(334) 242-3952

Alaska
Dept. of Health and Social Services
State of Alaska
240 Main Street, Suite 701
Juneau, AK 99811
(907) 465-2071

Arizona
Office of Substance Abuse
   Services/GMH
2122 East Highland
Phoenix, AZ 85016
(602) 553-9092

Arkansas
Bureau of Alcohol and
   Drug Abuse Prevention
Department of Health
5800 West 10th Street, Suite 907
Little Rock, AR 72204
(501) 280-4501

California
Department of Alcohol and
   Drug Programs
1700 K Street, 5th Floor
Sacramento, CA 95814-4037
(916) 445-1943

Colorado
Alcohol & Drug Abuse Division
Department of Human Services
4055 South Lowell Boulevard
Denver, CO 80236-3120
(303) 866-7480

Connecticut
Department of Mental Health &
   Addiction Services
410 Capitol Avenue, 4th Floor
Hartford, CT 06134
(860) 418-6958

Delaware
Alcohol & Drug Services
Agency of Health & Social Services
1901 N. DuPont Highway
New Castle, DE 19720
(302) 577-4461, Ext.46

Florida
Substance Abuse
Dept. of Children & Families
1317 Winewood Blvd
Building 3, Room 105
Tallahassee, FL 32399-0700
(850) 487-2920

Georgia
GA Department of Human Resources
Division of Mental Heath and
   Substance Abuse
Two Peachtree Street, NW
Suite 23202
Atlanta, GA 30303-3171
(404) 657-2273

Hawaii
Alcohol & Drug Abuse Division
Department of Health
Kakuhihewa Building
601 Kamokila Boulevard, Rm. 360
Kapolei, HI 96707
(808) 692-7506

Idaho
Division/Bureau of Mental
Health & Substance Abuse Services
450 West State Street, 5th Floor
Boise, ID 83720-0036
(208) 334-4944

Illinois
Office of Alcoholism &
   Substance Abuse
Department of Human Services
100 West Randolph, Suite 5-600
James R. Thompson Center
Chicago, IL 60601
(312) 814-2291

Indiana
Division of Mental Health Family &
   Social Services Administration
402 W. Washington Street, Rm. W353
Indianapolis, IN 46204-2739
(317) 232-7845

Iowa
Division of Substance Abuse &
   Health Promotion
Lucas State Office Building
3rd Floor
Des Moines, IA 50319
(515) 281-4417

Kansas
Substance Abuse/Mental Health/
   Development Disorders
Credit Union 1 Building
610 SW 10th Street, 2nd Floor
Topeka, KS 66612
(785) 296-3773

Kentucky
Division of Substance Abuse
Department of Mental Health
100 Fair Oaks, 4E-D
Frankfurt, KY 40621
(502) 564-2880

Louisiana
Office of Addictive Disorders
Department of Health & Hospitals
1201 Capitol Access Road
BIN# 18, 4th Floor
Baton Rouge, LA 70802
(225) 342-6717

Maine
Office of Substance Abuse
AMHI Complex
Marquardi Building, 3rd Floor
159 State House Station
Augusta, ME 04333-0159
(207) 287-6342

Maryland
Alcohol & Drug Abuse
   Administration
201 West Preston Street, 4th Floor
Baltimore, MD 21201
(410) 767-6925

Massachusetts
Bureau of Substance Abuse Services
250 Washington Street, 3rd Floor
Boston, MA 02108-4619
(617) 624-5151 or 5300

Michigan
Bureau of Substance Abuse Services
MI Dept. of Community Health
320 S. Walnut Street
Lansing, MI 48913
(517) 335-0278

Minnesota
Chemical Dependency Program
Department of Human Services
444 Lafayette Road
St. Paul, MN 55155-3823
(651) 582-1846

Mississippi
Division of Alcohol & Drug Abuse
Robert E. Lee State Office Building
11th Floor
239 N. Lamar Street
Jackson, MS 39201
(601) 359-1288

Missouri
Division of Alcohol & Drug Abuse
1706 E. Elm Street
Jefferson City, MO 65101
(573) 751-9449

Montana
Chemical Dependency Bureau
Addictive and Mental
    Disorders Division
1400 Broadway, Room C118
Helena, MT 59620
(406) 444-3964

Nebraska
Drug Abuse & Addiction Services
Nebraska Health & Human Services
Folsom & W. Prospector Place
Lincoln Regional Center Campus
Building 14
Lincoln, NE 68509
(402) 471-2851, Ext. 5583

Nevada
Department of Human
    Services/Health Division
Bureau of Alcohol & Drug Abuse
505 E. King Street, Room 500
Carson City, NV 89701
(775) 684-4190

New Hampshire
Bureau of Substance Abuse Services
Department of Health and
    Human Services
105 Pleasant Street
Concord, NH 03301
(603) 271-6105

New Jersey
Division of Addiction Services
120 South Stockton Street, 3rd Floor
Trenton, NJ 08611
(609) 292-9068 or 7385

New Mexico
Behavioral Health Services Division
Harold Runnels Building
Room 3300 North
1190 St. Francis Drive
Santa Fe, NM 87501
(505) 827-2658

North Carolina
Substance Abuse Services
Department of Health & Human
    Resources
3007 Mail Service Center
Raleigh, NC 27699-3007
(919) 733-4670, ext. 231

Ohio
OH Department of Alcohol & Drug
    Addiction Services
Two Nationwide Plaza
280 N. High Street, 12th Floor
Columbus, OH 43215-2537
(614) 466-3445

Oregon
Office of Alcohol and
    Drug Abuse Programs
Human Resources Building
500 Summer Street, NE
Salem, OR 97310-1015
(503) 945-5763

Rhode Island
Division of Substance Abuse
14 Harrington Road
Barry Hall Building #52
Cranston, RI 02920-3080
(401) 462-2351

New York
Office of Alcoholism and
    Substance Abuse Services
1450 Western Avenue
Albany, NY 12203-3526
(518) 457-2061

North Dakota
Division of Mental Health &
    Substance Abuse Services
600 South 2nd Street, Suite #1E
Bismarck, ND 58504-5729
(701) 328-8922

Oklahoma
Substance Abuse Services
1200 Northeast 13, 2nd Floor
Oklahoma City, OK 73117-1022
(405) 522-3857

Pennsylvania
PA Department of Health
Bureau of Drug and
    Alcohol Programs
2635 Paxton Street
Harrisburg, PA 17111
(717) 783-8200

South Carolina
Department of Alcohol & Drug
    Abuse Services
3700 Forest Drive, Suite 300
Columbia, SC 29204
(803) 734-9520

South Dakota
Division of Alcohol and Drug Abuse
Hillsview Plaza
East Highway 34
c/o 500 East Capitol
Pierre, SD 57501-5070
(605) 773-3123

Texas
TX Commission on Alcohol and
    Drug Abuse
9001 North IH 35, Suite 105
Austin, TX 78753-5233
(512) 349-6601

Vermont
Office of Alcohol and
    Drug Abuse Programs
VT Department of Health
108 Cherry Street
Burlington, VT 05402
(802) 651-1550

Washington
Division of Alcohol and
    Substance Abuse
612 Woodland Square Loop, SE
Building C
Olympia, WA 98504
(360) 438-8078

Wisconsin
Bureau of Substance Abuse Services
    and Family Services
1 West Wilson Street, Room 434
Madison, WI 53707-7851
(608) 266-3719

Tennessee
Bureau of Alcohol and
    Drug Abuse Services
Cordell Hull Building, 3rd Floor
425 5th Avenue North
Nashville, TN 37219
(615) 741-1921

Utah
Division of Substance Abuse
120 North 200 West, Room 413
Salt Lake City, UT 84103
(801) 538-3939

Virginia
Office of Substance Abuse Services
Department of Mental Health
1220 Bank Street, 8th Floor
Richmond, VA 23219
(804) 786-3906

West Virginia
Office of Behavioral Health
State Capitol Complex
Building 6, Room B-717
Charleston, WV 25305
(304) 558-3618

Wyoming
Division of Behavioral Health
Substance Abuse Program
2300 Capitol Avenue
Cheyenne, WY 82002
(307) 777-6494

ADDITIONAL NETWORK RESOURCES

American Samoa
Department of Human Resources
American Samoa Government
P.O. Box 997537
Pago Pago, AS 96799
(011-684) 633-2696

Guam
Drug and Alcohol Treatment
  Services
Department of Mental Health &
  Substance Abuse
790 Gov. Carlos G. Camacho Road
Tamuning, GU 96911
(671) 647-5440, 5325

Republic of Palau
Ministry of Health
Republic of Palau
P.O. Box 6027
Koror, Republic of Palau PW 96940
(011-680) 488-2552

District of Columbia
Addiction, Prevention and
  Recovery Administration
Department of Human Services
1300 First Street, NE, Suite 300
Washington, DC 20002
(202) 727-9393

Puerto Rico
Mental Health & Anti-Addiction
  Services Administration
Department of Health
Barbosa Avenue
Lincoln Bldg., #414 6th Floor
San Juan, PR 00928-1414
(787) 764-3670

Virgin Islands
VI Division of Mental Health
Alcoholism and Drug Dependency
  Services
Barbel Plaza South, 2nd Floor
St. Thomas, VI 00802
(340) 774-4888

NOTES

Chapter 1:

1. Virginia Ross, "Picking Up the Pieces," *Insight Magazine* (Ridgeview Institute) 19, no. 2 (Fall 1998).

2. Floyd Garrett, Behavioral Medicine Association, www.bma-wellness.com.

3. Kevin Lynch, "Prescription Addiction Can be a Most Insidious Threat," *Detroit News*, 5 August 1997, Metro section.

4. "Household Survey on Drug Abuse," Substance Abuse Mental Health Services Administration, 1999.

5. Greg Beaubien, "Lethal and Legal: Rampant Prescription Drug Abuse is America's Unnoticed Killer," *Detroit News,* 12 August 1996.

Chapter 4:

1. *American Journal of Psychiatry*, 1998.

2. Timothy McCall, M.D., "Should You Fire Your Doctor?" *Redbook* (October 2000): 49.

3. Jamie Court and Francis Smith, *Making a Killing: HMOs and the Threat to Your Health* (Monroe, Maine: Common Courage Press, 1999).

4. "Medicine Use Statistics," National Council on Patient Information and Education, www.talkaboutrx.org, 2000.

Chapter 5:
1. *Alive and Free* (Hazelden Foundation), September 27, 2000.
2. Gerhard Meyer, et. al., "Casino Gambling Increases Heart Rate and Salivary Cortisol In Regular Gamblers," *Biological Psychiatry* 48, no. 9 (1 November 2000): 948-953.
3. Lynda Hurst, "Why High Achievers Sometimes Risk All for Sex Addiction," *Toronto Star*, 15 January 2000, Saturday Edition 1, p. 15.
4. Rita Baron-Faust, "The Anatomy of Addiction: Are You At Risk?" *Cosmopolitan* (June 1990): 220.
5. *Diagnostic & Statistical Manual of Mental Disorders 4th Edition* (Washington, D.C.: American Psychiatric Association, 1994).
6. *PR Newswire* 21 (June 1996): 130
7. Steven M. Lynn, "Dual Diagnosis," *Insight Magazine* (Ridgeview Institute) 14, no. 2 (Fall 1993).
8. Information Services, Center For Substance Abuse Prevention (Washington, D.C.: U.S. Department of Health & Human Services).
9. Jennifer L. Rodgers, "Dual Diagnosis Issue Stirs Turf Fight Between Providers," *Eastern Pennsylvania Business Journal* 8, no. 2 (13 July 1997): 12.
10. Mary Jo Wich, "Pioneering Dual Diagnosis Care at St. Anthony's Medical Center," *Behavioral Health Management* 14, no. 2 (1994): 38.

Chapter 8:
1. Virginia Ross, "Picking Up the Pieces."
2. *Alcohol & Addiction Magazine* 12, no. 2 (March 1992): 13.
3. Virginia Ross, "Picking Up the Pieces.
4. Ibid.
5. Nan H. Davis, "International Pharmacists Anonymous," *Journal of Pharmacy* 4, no. 6 (1991): 362-368.

Chapter 10:
1. Kalpana Srinivasan, "Women's Hidden Addiction Reported," *Seattle Times*, 4 June 1998, Health & Science section.

Epilogue:
1. Donald R. Wesson and David E. Smith, "Prescription Drug Abuse-- Patient, Physician and Cultural Responsibilities," *Western Journal of Medicine*, 152 (May 1990): 613-616. Reprinted with permission of BMJ Publishing Group and Donald R. Wesson.